ACADEMIA TO BIOTECHNOLOGY: CAREER CHANGES AT ANY STAGE

· · · · · · · · · ·

ACADEMIA TO BIOTECHNOLOGY: CAREER CHANGES AT ANY STAGE

··········

Jeffrey M. Gimble

ELSEVIER
ACADEMIC
PRESS

AMSTERDAM • BOSTON • HEIDELBERG • LONDON
NEW YORK • OXFORD • PARIS • SAN DIEGO
SAN FRANCISCO • SINGAPORE • SYDNEY • TOKYO

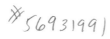

Elsevier Academic Press
200 Wheeler Road, 6th Floor, Burlington, MA 01803, USA
525 B Street, Suite 1900, San Diego, California 92101-4495, USA
84 Theobald's Road, London WC1X 8RR, UK

This book is printed on acid-free paper. ⊗

Library of Congress Cataloging-in-Publication Data
Application submitted

British Library Cataloguing in Publication Data
A catalogue record for this book is available from the British Library

ISBN: 0-12-284151-4

For all information on all Academic Press publications
visit our Web site at www.books.elsevier.com

PRINTED IN THE UNITED STATES OF AMERICA
04　05　06　07　08　09　9　8　7　6　5　4　3　2　1

To Josie and Gil

Contents

PREFACE

When I trained as a medical and graduate student, I thought I would spend my career pursuing research in a traditional academic setting; however, life is what happens while you are making other plans. The relationship between academia and the biotech industry changed. After spending 12 years as a faculty member in a nonprofit research foundation and university medical center, I was ready for a change of scenery. I left the relatively safe environment of academia in 1999 to join a biotechnology start-up company. One thing led to another and I found myself involved in co-founding a new company focusing on the use of adipose-derived adult stem cells for tissue engineering applications. It was a great opportunity and one that allowed me to discover the ups and downs of biotech. While these ups and downs sometimes occur for scientific reasons, often they reflect the enthusiasm (or lack thereof) and venture capital available in the marketplace. In the course of my four years in the biotech sector, I was exposed to a wide range of scientific, business, and management situations. While there was nothing I had not heard before, the firsthand experience gave me a different appreciation of the information. Before I decided to return to an academic position, I thought I would try to commit my impressions to print. I have the conceited idea that I actually learned a few things during my biotech years. Of course, nothing in this book is new, to me or to you; however, the associations I can draw might be of value to students and investigators who are considering which path to follow in a scientific career. Those who read the book will have a chance to see how I have organized my experiences into a practical guideline that can be used by a wide range of individuals at different career levels. Graduate students considering a career in biotech might use it to determine what skills their future employers will be looking for. Academics might find use for some of the organizational elements as they train their students. Alternatively, they might use it themselves if they embark on a transition to the biotech industry. Finally, scientists and administrators in biotech might use this book as an introductory training tool for new employees.

In a nutshell, here is what I discovered: There are many differences between what I will call academia and the biotechnology industry. There are also many similarities. While I thought I already knew this before leaving the university, my understanding was theoretical at best. I needed to work on both sides of the equation to appreciate what these differences and similarities meant in practice. On the surface, there are some tasks that are done better in a university laboratory and some that are more suited to an industry environment. For example, some people believe that creative work flourishes best in academia while product development is better suited to an industry setting. My conclusion is, yes and no. Rather than look at these as "either/or" situations, I have concluded that it is more productive to take a more inclusive "both/and" view. To prepare students for the challenges that we will all face in the decades ahead, scientific education needs to integrate the strengths and processes of both academia and industry into its training programs. I am not trying to predict what the future will be for any individual student; instead, I want to highlight and identify the common tools and skills that all people will need, regardless of the career paths they choose (or that choose them!).

ACKNOWLEDGMENTS

Once upon a time I thought that the two- or three-page acknowledgment sections in books I read were excessively long. Now that I am writing my own book, I appreciate that they were probably too short. I want to list at least some of the many people who have contributed to this work (and I apologize in advance to those of you who I left out!).

At Zen-Bio, Inc. (Research Triangle Park, NC), I thank my colleagues and associates Dawn Franklin, Renee Lea-Currie, PhD, Nicole Perkins, Arden Bond, and Peter Pierracini. At Artecel Sciences (Durham, NC), I thank my co-founders Bill Wilkison, PhD and Yuan-Di Halvorsen, PhD, without whom I would not have gained the experiences described here; the research staff, Anindita Sen, PhD, Bentley Cheatham, PhD, Blythe Devlin, PhD, Sandra Foster, PhD, Tracey du Laney, PhD, Kevin Hicok, MS, Amy Kloster, Dan Willingmyre, and Laura Aust for the opportunity to lead their efforts; and Bill Franklin, for exposing me to the nuances of the manufacturing process and regulatory affairs. At Cognate Therapeutics (Sunnyvale, CA and Baltimore, MD), I thank Ken Moseley, JD and Alan Smith, PhD for reviewing the chapters on patents and good practices. At Merchant & Gould (Atlanta, GA), I thank Joe Bennett-Paris, JD, PhD, for providing my introductory course on patent law and reviewing the chapter on patents and intellectual property. At The Southern Research Institute, I thank Vince Torti, PhD for reviewing the chapter on good practices. At Northern Illinois University, I thank Diane Gimble Johns, PhD, for reviewing the initial outline and selected chapters. At Duke University, I thank Farshid Guilak, PhD, Beverly Fermor, PhD, and all the members of the Orthopedic Research Division for their comments, suggestions, and critiques during the development of this book. At the Pennington

Biomedical Research Center (Baton Rouge, LA), I thank Ken Eilertsen, PhD for reviewing the chapters on closing a company, Anne Jarrett, JD for reviewing the chapters on patents and intellectual property, Gail Kilroy and Gena Doucet for reviewing the chapters related to human resource management, and Jennifer Rood, PhD for reviewing the chapters on closing and opening a lab.

I owe special thanks to two people:

Thomas Griggs, PhD, at New Science Consultants (Raleigh, NC) provided me with one-on-one hands-on leadership and management training. Anything I have to say about those subjects throughout the book, and especially in Chapter 23, "Personal Development," is simply my paraphrasing of his teachings; I only take credit for any mistakes that might be included in my text.

This book would never have been written without the opportunities, encouragement, and support provided to me by Carolyn Underwood, former President and CEO of Artecel Sciences (Durham, NC). I learned more about business and leadership under stress from Carolyn than anyone else I have worked with.

Finally, I owe my greatest thanks to Xiying and Jesse Wu, my wife and son. Without their help, I would have taken an entirely different path during this period of my career and never would have appreciated how much you can learn from a six-year-old mind.

1

· · · · · · · · · ·

COMMUNICATION

· · · · · · · · · · · · · · · · ·

In many ways, science is all about communication. Discoveries that remain hidden in laboratory notebooks might as well never have been made. You need to transmit your ideas and results to colleagues and peers through a variety of formal and informal media, including manuscripts, reports, and oral presentations. This chapter discusses how communication skills can improve your scientific career in both academia and biotechnology.

NONVERBAL

In the course of your career, you may have mastered the difficult art of how to communicate with others. If so, congratulations! Events in daily life continue to prove the inaccuracy of this conclusion for many individuals. Communication takes place on various levels and in different forms. The vast majority of it happens without a word (written, spoken, or otherwise). Nonverbal cues account for 70% or more of our communication. How you look at someone, how you walk, what you wear, how you smell, and where you sit or stand can all be interpreted and given meaning. For example, as a laboratory manager, you can get a very different response from your staff if you show up wearing a suit and tie than if you wear blue jeans and a tee shirt. The suit and tie might help you communicate better if you need to meet with the entire research team in an organizational meeting; the blue jeans and tee shirt might be more valuable if you need to meet individually with a graduate student or postdoctoral fellow. Even before you open your mouth in either circumstance, what people see will influence how they respond to what you have to say.

More importantly, it will influence what they hear when you say it. If you wear a suit and tie to a meeting with colleagues who find that clothing intimidating, their automatic response might be to see you as a potential threat. It would probably be difficult for them to hear you praise their progress and research activities because that praise could be misinterpreted as criticism.

Likewise, if you schedule an all-hands laboratory meeting to reorganize laboratory procedures in response to infractions noted by the organization's radiation safety inspectors and then show up in jeans and a tee shirt, you have just made your job a great deal more difficult. By "dressing casually," you are sending the message that the subject of the meeting is not important. Of course, it *is* important; if the laboratory does not correct itself, you may lose your privilege to use radioactivity in experiments for a year. And, as a leader, you need to use whatever forms of communication you can to get that point across.

Everyone uses common nonverbal communication cues, such as rolling eyes, slouching, shrugging, clenching fists, making body contact, frowning, smiling, crying, and laughing. Some of these cues are more obvious than others and represent different extremes of emotion. What sometimes may slip past your attention is that everyone has his or her own repertoire of nonverbal vocabulary that they use in "speech" every day. You may need to watch yourself on a video to fully appreciate the depth of your vocabulary. Once you see yourself in action, you may gain a better understanding of how you communicate through nonverbal cues and how this influences the way people respond to you on a daily basis.

VERBAL

Oral

Everyone is trained to use speech as early as possible. One of the major milestones in child rearing is baby's first word. Because speaking is fundamental to daily activity, many college programs in the sciences assume that it is a skill students have already mastered. It is less common today than it was two or three generations ago for public speaking to be a requirement in many college curricula. However, some scientific graduate training programs recognize that students need formal training in oral presentations. To address this, they require students to give a minimum number of seminars to an audience of faculty, students, and staff before graduation. After each presentation, students receive an evaluation of their performance and suggestions for improvement.

With practice, you can improve your speaking skills. More than anything else, self-confidence is critical for success. Nervous behaviors, such as inappropriate giggling, a quaking voice, or abject fear, will detract from your oral presentation. Other factors that determine your success include thought organization, language choice, and audience identification.

Public speaking takes place in different forums. In a seminar setting, you have the opportunity to prepare in advance, to develop audiovisual aids, and to set out a logical argument for your audience. In one-on-one interaction, speech is less formal and more interactive. Just as important as what you say is what you hear. If you fail to listen carefully with both your ears and your eyes, you risk misunderstanding what someone is saying to you, and similarly, you may fail to recognize when they misunderstand you. In a conversation, you need to pay attention to others' nonverbal cues to be sure that they are engaged with you and to assess whether information is accurately transmitted. If you receive input that they have failed to understand your statements, you need to backtrack and rephrase yourself. For example, suppose you are attending a fund-raising event for your scientific institution. A donor from the community without a scientific background asks you about your work. You will need to present your research in simple language without appearing condescending. One way to do this is to start out with a few background statements, and then ask your listener if what you have just said makes sense. It may be necessary to keep reengaging the donor with questions to determine how well you have communicated. If you do your job well, the donor will spontaneously ask you questions through your dialogue, providing direct input as to his or her degree of comprehension. And, if you are really successful, the institution will meet or exceed its fund-raising goals.

Written

In science, you will need to communicate on paper and electronically. Publications remain an important form of currency in academia and in industry. Your writing skills will be used in generating internal memos, standard operating procedures, test reports, business summaries, manuscripts for publication, and grant and patent applications. You can follow a generalized format for each of these specialized documents (to be described in later sections). Before setting out to write, it is always wise to prepare a detailed outline of the document's content. Taking the extra time up front to organize your thoughts will improve your efficiency in the long run. The first time you write a grant or peer-reviewed manuscript, it will

Table 1.1 *Public Speaking: Preparation for a Talk*	
Questions to Ask Yourself	*Steps to Prepare*
Who will be in my audience?	Ask the meeting organizer in advance about the make-up of your audience.
What material do I want to cover?	Organize your material (e.g., Introduction, Methods, Results, Discussion, Conclusion, Future Directions). Tell the audience how the talk will be organized before you start. Make sure you have a story to tell, even if you do not know what the ending is yet.
What are the critical messages I want to transmit to the audience?	Prepare PowerPoint slides if you will have a projector at your disposal. Do not hesitate to make slides with simple statements. Use the slides as memory aids for your presentation. Introduce each slide, tell the audience what is on it, and then summarize it before moving on to the next slide. People need to hear things multiple times and see reinforcing visual cues to assimilate new data.
How long should I talk?	Present a body of material consistent with the length of the talk. A common mistake is to try to cram a 45-minute talk into a 15-minute presentation. You will not convey more information by talking faster; the opposite is more likely! Try and leave a few minutes at the end for questions.
What is my worst-case scenario? The most common problems faced are:	
a. The audiovisual system malfunctions (no slides or no microphone).	a. One option may be to use a blackboard to present your ideas. It never hurts to have a good joke to tell under such circumstances.
b. A member of the audience interrupts you repeatedly with questions during your talk, derailing the logic, organization, and flow of your talk.	b. Never argue with a question from the audience. To gain time, always praise the quality of the question. Try to answer it as directly as possible and always stay to the point.
c. Your slides are out of order.	
d. You lose your voice.	Determine if you have provided the

(Continued)

Table 1.1	*Public Speaking: Preparation for a Talk (Continued)*
	information the questioner sought before moving ahead. Be prepared for further questions from the audience after you have been interrupted a first time; other members of the audience will be less inhibited thereafter.
	c. Practice shuffling the slides in your presentation and then giving the talk for each slide individually.
	d. Keep a glass of water on the podium when you speak.
What if I get stage fright?	Prepare an index card with the first few lines of the opening statement you want to make. Use the card as a back-up tool to help you get started. (Beginners may want to write out the entire talk and have a scripted speech; however, a talk will sound more natural if you speak spontaneously rather than read it.) Practice your talk in the empty auditorium or room in advance. Recruit friends and colleagues to critique your talk before presentation. Modify in response to their comments and repeat. During the actual talk, identify individuals in the audience and pretend you are talking to them alone.

appear to be an insurmountable hurdle. By reducing it to its components in an outline, you begin to make the task more manageable. Again, practice helps. The more frequently you write, the more facile you will become. No matter what you do, you will make your professional career infinitely easier if you refine and improve your writing skills.

When you write, your objective is to influence the reader's thoughts. Ultimately, your document must be informative, compelling, and persuasive. Some of the tools of newspaper writing will help you do this. Tell the reader the "who, what, where, why, and when" of your story in the opening paragraphs. Keep your sentences direct and in the active form. Avoid the past tense and passive voice. Sloppy writing will quickly lose the support of your reader. When readers encounter grammatical or spelling mistakes in your writing, they begin to wonder about your ability to pay attention to detail. If your reader is reviewing your grant application for a National Institutes of Health-funded, 5-year proposal with a budget of $1.5 million, you do not want him or her to be thinking about grammatical errors.

Listening

Almost anyone can benefit from a class on how to listen effectively. Like writing and speaking, listening is a skill that can be trained and developed. In part, listening relies on the same skills you use in speaking. You need to pay attention to your audience and take the time to hear what they are say-ing at multiple levels. When you meet with colleagues, you may listen for the comments you want or expect to hear in response to your questions. Take the extra effort to understand the things you did not want to hear in their answers. In the same way, state your questions carefully and leave them open-ended. Asking a supervisee if a project will be completed by a particular date is different than asking when a particular project will be completed. With the first question, you may get the answer you *want* to hear, but the second question may elicit the answer you *need* to hear. It is important to keep in mind that listening is not a passive process. You need to actively filter and store the information you receive. Remember, people who listen more (and speak less) in negotiations are more likely to achieve their objectives.

ORGANIZATION

Structure

All organizations develop some degree of structure. In part, the structure of an organization facilitates and accelerates communication among its members. This has the potential to reduce the time needed to accomplish repeated or similar tasks. Communication does not occur in a vacuum. Our society has structures designed to facilitate communication between indi-viduals. For example, when you purchase food in the grocery store, you and the checker both have preconditioned roles to play. You expect to dis-cuss the cost of items in your grocery cart and whether they should be placed in a plastic or paper bag. While communication can be limited to simple yes or no responses, it does not preclude discussion of the latest movies, your families, or other issues. Nevertheless, the content must focus on the commercial transaction and its completion. Otherwise, the remaining people in line will begin to express their opinions on why you are moving too slowly.

Similar structures and roles exist within scientific institutions. In part, this organizational structure defines responsibility and accountability. As a graduate student or postdoctoral fellow, you enter into a relationship with a faculty advisor/mentor. You accept certain responsibilities in the process to (1) conduct your research activities and generate data; (2) be a good citizen within the mentor's laboratory, assisting others in their work; (3) be fiscally conservative in ordering supplies and reagents; and (4) meet the requirements for graduation within your department. If you fail to accomplish these tasks, you are ultimately accountable for the outcome (no degree). At the same time, your mentor enters into a contract to: (1) provide an appropriately funded working environment for your training; (2) promote your scientific development and maturation; and (3) protect your welfare within the department and university.

By taking on a role in the relationship, you accept certain communication responsibilities. You report to your advisor or his or her designee on a regular basis. It is likely that you have developed a format to streamline and monitor your interactions. This might take the form of notes summarizing previous meetings and identifying points for further discussion or consideration. Each time you meet, you each have specific objectives that you wish to address. These will include particular scientific projects, their progress, future directions, graduation plans, and personal issues; one, two, or all of these topics may be on the agenda at any given meeting.

At the same time, you might also serve in a supervisory role within the laboratory's organization. For example, you may have been assigned to mentor a sophomore undergraduate working part-time in the laboratory. In this capacity, you must oversee and guide the student's activities on a regular basis. You become responsible for his or her progress and share credit for both successes and failures. Certain tools, such as lists, frequent meetings, and management techniques, can improve the odds for success.

Lists

It is difficult to manage multiple tasks, particularly those that rely on the input and participation of others. One way to deal with this issue is to generate and maintain a list. While you may have a good memory, you are not a computer (fortunately!).

Lists can be used for immediate and long-term tasks. For example, you may find it helpful to organize your day by writing down and prioritizing your scheduled activities (meetings, writing projects, experiments). Do this either at the end of the preceding day or first thing upon arriving in the office each morning. While you may not complete all of your "chores," this exercise will allow you to keep track of outstanding commitments. This same approach is valuable for long-range planning, especially for tasks involving a group of individuals. When initiating a project, it is prudent to define and record the objectives your team seeks to accomplish. These can include long-term aims (final goals) and milestones (identifiable points of achievement on the path to each goal). The next step in the process is to define the "action points" to be assigned to individual team members that are necessary for the completion of the project. These action points should include objective criteria documenting what constitutes an acceptable or unacceptable outcome for the endeavor. It is possible to use these criteria to define "go" or "no-go" decision points. Once these concepts are committed to a list, it should be circulated among the team members, reviewed, and revised as necessary. By building consensus among the team from the outset, you will have obtained commitment to a common goal and purpose. At future team meetings, this calendar of the task, its components, and the predetermined acceptance criteria provide a mechanism to track the progress of the overall project at interim time points. These tools will assist your team in reaching future decisions in a straightforward and relatively nonjudgmental manner.

Frequency of Meetings

It is better not to rely on chance encounters at the company coffee pot or in the hallway to maintain communication within a team or between individuals. Instead, it is more effective to establish and maintain a regular time for discussion. This can be done "one on one" between supervisors and supervisees or for an entire team or staff. By proactively determining a set time and agenda for meetings, you will improve the quality and timing of information transfer. Rather than meeting whenever a crisis arises, you may be able to avoid problems altogether.

You need to consider several factors when scheduling meetings. First, is one party fairly junior? If so, then the frequency should be adjusted to allow that individual both a degree of independence and easy access to supervision. While there is no need to micromanage, it is important to provide adequate guidance during early stages of development. The frequency of meetings can be reduced as an individual matures and he or she achieves greater autonomy. Alternatively, the meeting agenda can be advanced to a different plane to provide a new level of educational interaction.

Second, is one party in need of specific information on a regular basis? If you are meeting with your company's CEO to provide updates on a particular project, do it at regular intervals. Allow the CEO to have a full command of the project's scientific progress at all times. Your CEO may need to present to investors or corporate partners at any time, and he or she needs to be prepared. If your CEO does not have an advanced scientific degree, you may provide him or her with "on-the-job" scientific training. Treat the meetings as an opportunity to explain your research program in detail and to gain an ally for the future.

Third, what is appropriate to everyone's schedule? We all have too many meetings taking up our valuable time. Do not schedule any more meetings than you really need.

Managing up

When you meet with a supervisor, view the action as a dynamic opportunity. You are a participant and have control over the agenda. If possible, prepare an agenda for the meeting. Obtain agreement over tasks and objectives you hope to accomplish. Do not overextend your meeting in terms of time and content. Arrive prepared to deal with the issues you have included in your agenda. Be ready to present a plan for each task and a possible solution to potential problems. Most managers will appreciate an employee who takes a problem-solving approach; they prefer this to someone who simply arrives with a list of issues that need resolution.

Managing down

You need to be able to function on both sides of the "corporate" divide. Try to provide your supervisees with the same respect and empowerment you would desire in their position. Build a consensus in identifying the shared tasks and objectives of your team. Allow your team members to participate as much as possible in the planning phase of a project. By allowing the team to provide input, you facilitate their "buy in" to the overall objectives. Once the major goals are identified, give the team the freedom to work out the nitty-gritty details; let them decide on the interim milestones necessary to reach the final goals. I look for team players whose skills are better than my own; they might be able to run gels, culture cells, or isolate proteins more efficiently than I do. So, it makes sense to let them determine the steps in accomplishing those particular tasks. For many scientists, this process of letting go is one of the hardest steps to take. Most of our training from undergraduate to postdoctoral fellowship rewards us for doing everything ourselves. Breaking this pattern of behavior takes a conscious effort.

Once all the steps in a project's plan are laid out, be sure to review the plan with all parties concerned and then commit it to record. You should implement the experiment or process only after reaching this point. You may feel that the process outlined above is inefficient and time consuming. After you and your colleagues gain practice, it will go quicker and you will see benefits in terms of morale, productivity, and successful outcomes.

chapter

2

· · · · · · · · · ·

INTERFACING WITH SIBLING DEPARTMENTS

· · · · · · · · · · · · · · · · ·

A biotechnology company is an amalgam of diverse subcultures (Table 2.1). Each arena has its own viewpoint and priorities. This chapter compares the responsibilities of several biotech subcultures. There is a continuum existing within the organization among these subcultures in which the idea or product is passed along in an assembly line fashion.

BIOTECH SUBCULTURES

Research

Many academic life scientists fit most comfortably into the world of *research*. Here, the ideal focus is on "basic" science with an emphasis on mechanistic, hypothesis-driven experiments exploring the cutting edge of a question.

Development

Once *research* identifies a potential scientific application, *development* translates the idea into practice by providing "proof-of-principle" data to

Table 2.1   *Biotech Subcultures*
Research
Development
Manufacturing and Quality Control/Assurance
Clinical/Medical
Accounting/Business Development/Marketing
Legal

further direct the process. This involves greater emphasis on reproducibility, reliability, and documentation of the data rather than on discovery.

Manufacturing and Quality Control/Assurance

This department may be involved in scaling up the scientific operation, such as cell culture or protein production. Often, such steps rely on the expertise of a chemical or biochemical engineer. The focus here is to define matters in absolute terms, possibly in the form of a mathematical equation. The intent is to reduce the scientific hypothesis into an absolute certainty with 100% reproducibility, independent of the scientific operator or practitioner. There is no room for error or deviation from established protocols. The focus is to meet the demands of the regulatory and commercial environment outside the confines of the company.

Clinical/Medical

This department is concerned with physician and patient acceptance of the ultimate product. Its intent is to provide the medical consumer(s) with an easy to use and affordable service. Even if you discover the most advanced biomaterial for fracture repair, orthopedic surgeons will not welcome it if it requires a significant deviation from and lengthy extension of their standard operating room practices.

Accounting/Business Development/Marketing

These personnel will always focus on the bottom-line dollar. No scientific discovery can be supported if it will not lead to a commercially successful product for the company. This means that the research costs cannot be greater than the potential revenue within a reasonable amount of time. It does not pay to spend $600 million to develop a single product when its predicted annual market value is $20 million. Marketers must estimate how much a scientific discovery is worth based on the price the consumer is willing to pay. The health care industry has unofficial "threshold amounts" for particular procedures and diseases. For some diseases, a product with a price exceeding $1,000 will not be viable, whereas for others, the threshold may be 10–20 times higher. This reflects the severity of the disease, the cost of treatment and hospitalization based on existing modalities, and the presence (or absence) of third party payers.

Legal

The *legal* arm of the company will focus on scientific issues relating to intellectual property. It will pursue the following questions with you routinely: If you make a novel discovery, can you patent the information? Have you infringed on existing patents in the course of making your discovery? If so, do you need to obtain a license from the current patent holder to generate your product?

Summary

A company must bring these diverse viewpoints into focus around a common goal. Each of the company's subcultures uses what it considers to be objective criteria to reach a decision. For someone trained in a different discipline, it may be difficult to appreciate this fact. As a scientist, this means you must begin to reach or accept decisions with the input of "non-scientific" factors. This can be a challenge. Nevertheless, if any one of the constituent subcultures within a company is ignored, the outcome is more likely to be everyone's failure rather than success. Working within a biotech company will require compromises by all parties. This is not to imply that you will compromise the integrity or accuracy of the science itself, but only that you will face decisions in which a product will not be pursued for good reasons, despite the presence of good science. In the best of all worlds, the staff within each of the biotech's subcultures will reach a mutual understanding and respect for each other's expertise as well as the importance of their contribution to achieving a successful product.

3

·········

THE CIRCULAR CONTINUUM: PAPERS TO GRANTS TO PATENTS

················

In both academia and biotechnology, writing skills are of critical importance. The ability to craft peer-reviewed publications, grants, and patents is an essential tool for success in the intellectual property (IP) continuum. In academia, papers carry the most importance, followed by grants and then patents. In biotech, however, patents take first priority, followed by papers and then grants. This chapter discusses each of these documents and focuses on efficient ways to integrate their design and completion.

MANUSCRIPTS

A manuscript in a peer-reviewed journal is the fundamental monetary unit in science. Your publications make up your permanent, public record of accomplishment. The first writing project many of us faced in our scientific careers involved the reporting of our work in manuscript format. The ability to accumulate high quality, novel information and to present it in a clear and logical manner is essential both in academia and the biotech industry.

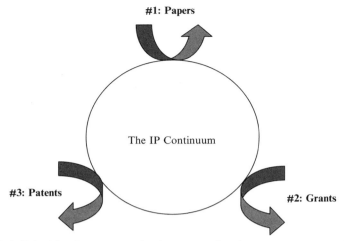

Figure 3.1 Priorities from an academic perspective: how to report your data.

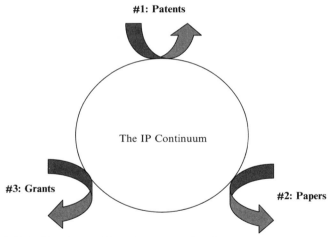

Figure 3.2 Priorities from a biotech perspective: how to maximize return on your intellectual property.

No matter where you go, data talks. Once written, a manuscript can serve this function in multiple ways. First, it communicates to the public the information that your scientific team has developed. In addition to other scientists, this public includes investors, business analysts, and venture capitalists interested in the biotech arena. Second, the format of a manuscript provides the basis for potential grant applications. The publication lends credibility to your laboratory's competence and the direction of your future research. It improves the likelihood that granting agencies will respond favorably to your requests for funding. Third, the manuscript is a springboard to patent applications. The methods and results contained in the manuscript will become the examples and background supporting your patent's claims. Finally, the manuscript's figures and text provide you with everything you will need to make oral presentations of your work in both scientific and business forums. Chapter 4 will discuss the strategy of preparing a manuscript.

GRANTS

Whether you are in academia or business, you will need money to support your research. Researchers in universities and not-for-profit institutions routinely submit grant applications to the federal government and private research foundations for funding. The private sector is also eligible for grant support. Annually, 2.5% of the federal research budget is specifically set aside for Small Business Innovative Research (SBIR) grants (http://grants.nih.gov/grants/funding/sbirsttr_programs.htm). In addition, at least 0.3% of the federal research budget is earmarked for the Small Business Technology Transfer (STTR) program. Companies with less than 500 employees are eligible to apply for these funds. The two programs differ in that companies applying for STTR funds must do so in collaboration with a university or not-for-profit research center. While the principal investigator on an STTR may be a university employee, the principal investigator on an SBIR must be an employee of the company. For-profit companies can also apply for government contracts in response to specific agency requests for research or service.

Many experienced scientists believe that the best grants are those for which 90% of the work has already been completed. Successful grant applications to the National Institutes of Health (NIH) and other federal agencies generally share features in common. Some of these are considered below:

1. They are traditionally *hypothesis* driven. Grant reviewers want you to demonstrate that your studies will provide an unambiguous answer to a defined question. Independent of the outcome, the study must provide useful information that will advance your field of science.
2. Grants are *focused*. Reviewers will want you to narrow the scope of your studies. Studies that are too broad are rejected as "diffuse and unfocused."
3. The ideas and specific aims of the grant are laid out in a logical progression. The grant must convey the necessary background, preliminary

data, and experimental design of its studies in an easy-to-read manner. If you force the reviewer to extrapolate or interpret your ideas, you are already losing ground.

4. The grant contains identifiable milestones with decision tree formats explaining how you will direct your research efforts in response to unknown future data. The milestones include quantifiable metrics suitable for statistical evaluation.

Chapter 5 will discuss the strategy of preparing a grant application.

PATENTS

Although a manuscript may be the basic monetary unit of science, it is the equivalent of a charitable donation from a business perspective if your intellectual property does not have patent protection. A patent gives you the right to prevent someone from practicing a novel tool or method you have invented. To be eligible for patenting, you cannot have made your idea freely available to the public. Any of the following constitutes a public disclosure of your idea: posters or oral presentations at meetings, invited talks, letters to colleagues, and publications. The date of a disclosure occurs when the information hits the streets; if your poster abstract appears electronically online a month before the actual meeting, that becomes the disclosure date. While the U.S. Patent Office allows investigators to obtain patents on ideas for up to 12 months after a public disclosure, the majority of the world's legal systems do not.

There are two general strategies to consider for patent applications:

1. Retroactive approach: In this scenario, you will submit patent applications only after you have completed all of the experiments required to fully support and document your idea. The advantage to this approach is that it reduces the risk to the institution. Now an internal team of scientific and legal advisors can evaluate the data to answer the important questions: will a patent be granted and, if so, will it have value to the institution? The retroactive approach has certain disadvantages. First, it delays the priority date of the final patent application; if anyone else has filed a similar idea, he or she may interfere with your final patent application even if you have more substantial data in your application. Second, it requires discipline by you and members of your team. Any unauthorized public disclosure of your data can jeopardize your patent application. The longer you wait to file, the risk increases that an inadvertent conversation or presentation will take place. If you absolutely

must talk about a project to an investor group or other institution, you need to formalize the process with a signed *confidential disclosure agreemen* (CDA). You will discover that this legal convention can be burdensome, particularly when working with large companies where the scientific and legal arms are not in close proximity or daily communication.

2. Proactive approach: In this scenario, you will submit a provisional patent application upon the inception of an idea. The advantage of this approach comes down to speed. It ensures that the patent office will award you the earliest possible priority date. It demarcates your "turf" in the intellectual property arena. The likelihood of an inadvertent public disclosure becomes a moot point, and the restrictions on scientific discussions are reduced. There are drawbacks. Without fully developing your idea in the laboratory prior to filing, it is possible that you will poorly or incorrectly present your idea, thereby jeopardizing your claims. Your final data may uncover additional intellectual property, and your original patent application may compromise your ability to claim this new territory. Indeed, your further experiments may fail to support your patent claims altogether, and the entire application will prove to be a waste of legal resources and filing fees.

Despite these risks, the proactive approach for patent filings is recommended for one reason alone: timing! Timing is critical. You have more to lose by filing late than by filing early. Your legal counsel will be able to assist you in this process. I recommend that scientists learn to communicate effectively with their patent attorneys and technology transfer officers. They have a great deal of information to teach you. Likewise, you can make their job easier by drafting the initial version of the patent. This will translate the science into a format they can readily understand and will reduce the preparation costs substantially. This will be discussed in Chapter 6.

REVIEWING

Journal editors and granting agencies will eventually call on you to help review your peers' manuscripts and grant applications. Reviewing will teach you more about what makes a manuscript or grant application strong (and what does not). A few words of advice about reviewing: remember the Golden Rule and do unto others as you would have them do unto you. Most of the time, the tendency is to do unto others as you *think* has been done to you. Try to keep a positive focus when evaluating grants and manuscripts; keep in mind the amount of effort that the investigator has put into the proposal. First, identify those aspects of the work that you support and state your appreciation of it. When pointing out areas for improvement or in error, keep your comments constructive, objective, and without personal bias. If you ever find yourself in a position where there is the potential appearance of a conflict of interest, recuse yourself from the review process. If you are uncertain about conflict of interest matters, bring the issue to the attention of the editor or program administrator and allow him or her to make the final judgment. Take the opportunity to serve as a reviewer whenever it arises. You will learn something from the experience (and there is always more to learn!). More and more, editors and program administrators are having difficulty in recruiting qualified reviewers. You will be serving the scientific community at large by agreeing to take on this task.

4

••••••••••

DESIGNING A MANUSCRIPT

••••••••••••••••••

The art of manuscript writing is something that continues to evolve. A well-written paper published in a prestigious journal circa 1980 would not necessarily be acceptable today; however, this can be attributed to higher expectations concerning data content rather than to the writing style. The fundamentals of manuscript preparation have remained similar over time. This chapter discusses some of the basic themes you need to consider as you design and write manuscripts for peer-reviewed journals.

CONTENTS OF A MANUSCRIPT

The process of writing a manuscript serves multiple purposes. First, it is a mechanism to report your findings and progress to your scientific peers. Second, it teaches others in the field how to reproduce your findings. Third, it provides a public record of your professional accomplishments. And, most importantly, it is a tool that allows you to plan your experiments and identify where gaps might exist in your logic or in the content of your data. Manuscripts follow the pattern of the classical "scientific method" that you probably learned in your seventh grade science class.

There are several ways to pursue a manuscript. One is to "follow your nose" experimentally and see where your data will lead; this approach gives you the greatest opportunity for a serendipitous finding. Another is

Table 4.1 *Contents of a Manuscript*	
Section	*Purpose*
Background Information (Introduction)	What is the premise of your study? What information does a reader need to be aware of?
Hypothesis (Introduction)	What do you propose to test in your study?
Materials	What do you need to do your experiments? Where do you buy the reagents?
Methods	What are the protocols you follow in the experiments?
Results	What are your data? What are their statistical significance?
Conclusions (Discussion, Opening Paragraph)	What does your data tell you?
Discussion	How does your data fit into the existing body of literature? What will be the next stage of development in the study?

to conduct experiments and, after you accumulate the proverbial "least publishable unit" (five figures and a table), to write it up; this will achieve quantity if not quality in your curriculum vitae. A third approach is to choose a journal, evaluate the contents and layout of a representative paper, and model your own work in accordance with the journal's apparent guidelines.

A proactive approach using the scientific method to outline your entire manuscript in advance of the study is recommended. This approach does not require you to know the outcome of your experiments in advance, but it instead has you simply consider what possible outcomes you may encounter. This planning exercise can reveal potential pitfalls in your study design or alternative experimental approaches that will reduce costs in terms of time and money. The resulting outline for the final manuscript provides a blueprint on how to perform your experiments and gives you internal metrics for measuring your success. If 3 months go by and you have not been able to get past Figure 1, you may need to reevaluate your plan.

Designing a manuscript is less time consuming than you might think. Together with your colleagues, identify the question you wish to ask. At the same time, review the existing literature that both supports and contradicts the hypothesis you have proposed. Next, outline the experiments you need to perform in order to answer the hypothetical question. Be sure to consider the following:

1. Has anyone else already published essentially the same experiment? If so, you need to seriously reevaluate your experimental plans. If not, proceed to step 2.
2. What are the possible outcomes of the experiments?
3. How many times will you need to repeat individual experiments to achieve statistical significance?
4. What controls (both positive and negative) do you need to run in each experiment?
5. How will you present the results of these experiments (as a table, bar graph, photomicrograph, etc.)?
6. How many experiments will be required to support a positive or negative conclusion?

Develop a list of the "take home" messages you will be able to support with either a positive or negative outcome to your proposed experiments. This will serve as a basis for your final conclusions and discussion.

Consider each manuscript in the context of your laboratory's resources, focusing on people, time, and money. You are advised to coordinate completion of the manuscript with the timelines of your key personnel. For example, if the first author on your study is a senior student who is preparing to defend his or her thesis, try to get all of the manuscripts submitted prior to the student's graduation date. This way, if the journal reviewers request additional experiments prior to acceptance, you are positioned more favorably to meet their demands. It is more difficult to complete the writing of manuscripts (much less to perform further experiments) once a graduate student has moved out of your laboratory for postdoctoral training.

Each manuscript represents a significant allocation of financial resources. Take the time to evaluate whether the paper has paid for itself by calculating the salaries of the personnel involved, the supplies and reagents used, and the page charges from the journal; the latter can be substantial if your figures are in color. The expenses (and their sources) may surprise you. Whenever possible, a manuscript should serve the needs of your laboratory's existing grants by documenting your completion of a *specific aim* or of future grant applications by generating supportive preliminary data. The research within the manuscript should open doors to new research opportunities rather than lead to a "dead end."

Consider the audience and "impact factor" of the journals in which you would like to publish your manuscript. You should try to publish your work in a journal that will best reach the scientific community most closely involved with your research activities. If possible, try to publish in a journal that will also expose your work to investigators beyond your immediate field. One way to gauge whether a journal is widely read is through its impact factor. Thomson-ISI (http://www.isinet.com/) calculates each major scientific journal's impact factor annually based on the journal's past 2 years of performance, using the number of manuscripts published and the number of times the journal was cited. While there is significant debate in the scientific and academic community concerning the relevance of impact factors, you are advised to use this information in making your publishing decisions. Even if you do not, you can be assured that, at some point in your career (tenure review, promotion, job interview), your publication record will be evaluated in the context of its associated impact factors.

5

· · · · · · · · · ·

DESIGNING AND WRITING
A GRANT

· · · · · · · · · · · · · · · · ·

Your manuscript-writing experience will translate directly to your grant-writing tasks. The manuscript contents have a role to play in the context of your grants; however, grants also emphasize and include additional components. Grant writing is as much an art form as it is a science. Grants need to convey an energy and enthusiasm above and beyond that of a manuscript. This chapter discusses strategies to use in designing and writing your grants.

As both an art and a science, grant writing is a fundraising activity and, in a sense, a sales pitch. Without ever meeting the reviewers face to face, you need to convince them that you are:

1. Enthusiastic about your work
2. Productive
3. At an institution that can support the work
4. Knowledgeable in the relevant scientific field
5. Qualified to do the work as demonstrated by significant preliminary data
6. Have command of a clear and logical experimental design plan that will result in useful experimental data regardless of the outcome of your study
7. Are smart enough to know what to do if you run into problems
8. The best person to fund for the project

Table 5.1	*Components of a Grant*
Budget	How much will it really cost? Is the expense justifiable?
Curriculum Vitae	What are the credentials of the team working on the project?
Resources	Do you have the equipment to do the work?
Specific Aims (Goals)	What is your hypothesis? How do you plan to test it?
Background and Significance	What evidence supports your hypothesis? Why should anyone care about whether it is right or wrong?
Preliminary Data/Progress	What data have your laboratory generated on the subject?
Experimental Design	What is the detailed design of your experiments?
Commercialization Plan	What is the business model for how you will translate the science into a product? How soon will that happen?
Human Subjects Protection	Do you meet the federal regulatory requirements in your use of human subjects?
Experimental Animal Protection	Do you meet current veterinary standards in your use of experimental animals?
References	Do you acknowledge appropriate literature in your design (particularly any papers by potential reviewers)?
Collaborator/Consultant Support Documents	Do you document that you really have the collaborators listed in the application?

To accomplish this task, your writing needs to be persuasive, easy to read, and to the point. Although our training in science emphasizes facts and figures, grant writing calls for the skills we gained in freshman English and seminars with graded term papers. The reviewers are busy people and will be reading many applications in addition to your own. They will not appreciate errors in spelling or grammar, fuzzy writing, and excessive use of jargon and abbreviations. Flow charts, decision trees, and summary tables will help convey your message to the reviewer.

Who Is Your Target Audience?

You need to target your grant application to a specific agency or foundation. The formats you will use to write grants for the National Institutes of Health (NIH), the U.S. Department of Defense, or the National Institutes for Standards and Technology (NIST) are completely different. Be sure to study the granting agency's forms and regulations before proceeding with your outline. Visit the agency's web site for the most up-to-date information about its processes. You may be able to obtain the names of the individuals serving as peer reviewers (such information is available from the NIH in its Study Section Rosters). This information can help you tailor your application to the study section's area of expertise and focus.

Budget

A class in business accounting is something most scientists have never had in college (and many now wish that they did). While grant applicants tend to focus on the science, a grant is also about money. A grant that fails to pay the full cost of the project and is still expected to fully deliver on its promises creates problems at the end of the fiscal year. You need to demonstrate that the budget you have requested is appropriate for the outlined studies, and you also need to consider all the costs of the activity. In addition to salary for personnel, you must consider their fringe benefits. Your supply costs should include both the cost of the materials and the cost of shipping them to your facility. Be prepared to deal with the indirect costs factor covering the administration and overhead (rent, utilities, phones, mail, etc.) of your organization. Furthermore, take into account inflationary cost increases in goods and salaries during the future years of your grant. Although you may have accountants to assist you in developing your budget, the more you understand of the process, the better.

Curriculum Vitae

The grant application is only as good as the people involved. You need to provide documentation that you, your colleagues, and your collaborators have the expertise, training, and record of productivity required to successfully complete the project. Where you received your graduate and postgraduate training, what you have published, and what positions of responsibility you have held within the scientific community are all relevant. While this may seem like blowing your own horn, remember, no one else is going to do it for you.

RESOURCES

Study section members need to know that your laboratory and institution have the equipment, support staff, and core facilities required by the scientific project. You need to provide a detailed list describing your resources. Do not take anything for granted. For example, the study section will not assume that you have a particular piece of equipment even if your experimental design calls for it; make sure you list the specific item in the resources section of the application.

OUTLINE AND SPECIFIC AIMS

As you begin to write a grant, take the extra time to develop a detailed outline. The most important step is to define the *specific aims*, or goals, you wish to accomplish. Historically, granting agencies have favored grants that are "hypothesis-driven" rather than "descriptive" in nature. Reviewers favor applications that test a clearly defined hypothesis with a logical series of experiments yielding "yes/no" or "go/no-go" answers. With the recent development of methods evaluating the proteome and transcriptome, reviewers are more receptive to "information-driven" applications. The specific aims should be manageable in number. Grants listing five or more aims during a 3- to 5-year period will appear overly ambitious.

BACKGROUND AND SIGNIFICANCE

The intent of this section is to point the reviewer to the information in the literature relevant to your study. Even though you should not provide an extensive review of the literature, you need to demonstrate your command of the subject. It is wise to include the landmark papers in the field as references since it is likely that their authors will be involved in reviewing your proposal. It is important to link your specific aims directly to the background information. By the time the reviewer has read your background section, he or she should see how your experiments are going to fill in specific gaps in the existing knowledge base.

Preliminary Data

Granting agencies such as the National Institutes of Health (NIH) favor grants that include extensive preliminary data sections. Other agencies, such as the Defense Advanced Research Projects Administration (DARPA), are more receptive to projects at early stages of development. In the best of all worlds, your preliminary data section should include results relevant to each of your specific aims. On the other hand, if you present too much information, a reviewer will question whether there is anything of substance remaining to be done. You will need to balance how much data to include (never an easy decision). Some would argue that the best grant is one that is 90% completed and 100% unpublished. Unfortunately, the best guide for this process is experience and intuition.

Experimental Design

One way to approach this section is to consider each specific aim of the grant as a potential manuscript or manuscripts. In that context, use the tools outlined in Chapter 4 to define the experimental design section. Regardless of whether you are writing your grant from an academic or commercial institution, you will want to have the opportunity to report the work in the form of a peer-reviewed publication.

State a rationale for the specific study, and identify how it will address a particular hypothesis. Also, identify the materials and methods that will be employed. To simplify the transfer of information, reduce the design to a flowchart or diagram outlining the interrelation between experiments. Provide sufficient information and methodology to verify your competence to the reviewers. Define the metrics and statistical tools you will use to measure the success of your experiments. Discuss the possible outcomes you may achieve and how you will respond to each of them. Also demonstrate that you have considered the possible experimental pitfalls and have developed alternative strategies to deal with them. Provide a timeline for the completion of the various experiments. In addition, you need to publicly document your understanding of the resource and time allocation issues for the project. Most importantly, underpin your experimental design with an all-encompassing logic. There needs to be an unbreakable thread connecting each of your specific aims. For example, you should not design a study in which the initiation of Aim 2 is entirely dependent on a particular outcome in Aim 1. If you fail to make the expected observations in Aim 1, your design for Aim 2 no longer has relevance and jeopardizes your funding for the later years of the grant period.

COMMERCIALIZATION

For Small Business Innovative Research and Advanced Technology Projects, you will need to include a commercialization section in your grant. This needs to demonstrate how the science will be translated into a commercial project with a projected timeline for development, a market analysis of the potential consumer base, and an analysis of business competitors and partners. Much of this information should be available in the Business Plan of a biotechnology company. It needs to be formatted to meet the specifications of the granting agency. This section has particular benefit whenever you need to make a presentation to venture capitalists or other corporate investors/partners.

HUMAN AND ANIMAL SUBJECTS

No matter where you apply for funding, you will need to meet some level of oversight with respect to human and animal subjects. Each year, the regulations governing these issues become more sophisticated. For most work involving any living human subjects, either as patients or volunteers and including the use of test results, DNA analysis, or archival materials, you will need to submit the proposal to an Investigational Review Board (IRB). These panels are composed of physicians, academic scholars, community representatives, and ethicists who determine the legitimacy of the study and whether it adequately safeguards patients' rights. You can contact IRBs at local university medical schools or graduate schools, at major research hospital centers, or as private contractors. The IRB should be federally registered with the Department of Health and Human Services Office for Human Research Protections (OHRP). You will need to include documentation that your grant has been reviewed and approved by an accredited IRB before you can receive funding.

Similar restrictions apply to animal welfare. Research studies proposing to use animal subjects must be reviewed by an Institutional Animal Care and Use Committee (IACUC) composed of a veterinarian, scientist, ethicist, and community representative. These panels ensure that animals are used in accordance with the guidelines established by the Association for Assessment and Accreditation of Laboratory Animal Care (AAALAC) and other veterinary accreditation bodies. Investigators must document that they have explored all alternative testing models and are using the minimum number of test subjects necessary for their study. The IACUCs at universities and research institutions meet frequently (monthly) to review new experimental and grant application proposals. You will need to include documentation that your grant has been reviewed and approved by an accredited IACUC before you can receive funding.

REFERENCES

There will never be a grant that includes too many references, but there are many that leave out the critical ones. Science is never conducted in a vacuum, and it is important to acknowledge the sources of your information. Your references section will demonstrate your command of the literature and appreciation of the field's key contributors over the years.

CONSULTANTS OR COLLABORATORS

As the number and breadth of techniques in science expands, it is increasingly difficult for one laboratory to perform them all. If you recognize that your study faces a technical limitation, do not try to reinvent the wheel. Instead, identify and seek out a consultant or collaborator with the necessary expertise. Include his or her study in your budget as a consultant or subcontract/consortium cost, and formalize the relationship in the form of a letter from the collaborator; this should be included as a supplement to your grant application. Ultimately, the goal of the grant is not to train technicians in your laboratory but to answer the grant's hypothetical question. You should take the path of least resistance to reach this point.

REFERENCES

http://www.darpa.mil/baa/ Grants page for the Defense Advanced Research Projects Administration (DARPA).

http://www.science.doe.gov/grants/ Grants page for the Department of Energy.

http://grants1.nih.gov/grants/index.cfm Grants page for the National Institutes of Health (NIH).

http://www.nsf.gov/home/grants.htm Grants page for the National Science Foundation (NSF).

http://www.aaalac.org/position.htm Home page for the Association for Assessment and Accreditation of Laboratory Animal Care (AAALAC).

http://www.darpa.mil/ Home page for DARPA.

http://www.iacuc.org/ Home page for the Institutional Animal Care and Use Committee (IACUC).

http://www.nih.gov/ Home page for the NIH.

http://ohrp.osophs.dhhs.gov/irb/irb_guidebook.htm Web site for the Department of Health and Human Services Office of Human Research Protection (OHRP).

http://www.niaid.nih.gov/ncn/grants/default.htm Writing tips for National Institute for Allergy and Infectious Diseases (NIAID) grants.

http://grants.nih.gov/grants/grant_tips.htm Writing tips for NIH grants.

Reif-Lehrer, L. *Grant Application Writer's Handbook.* Boston: Jones & Bartlett Publishers, 1995.

6

· · · · · · · · · ·

DESIGNING AND WRITING
A PATENT

· · · · · · · · · · · · · · · · ·

Whether you are in academia or biotechnology, your intellectual property is valuable. Even if you do not intend to develop a product yourself, you should reserve this right for others by filing a patent protecting your invention or discovery. Without a patent, the likelihood that the idea can develop commercially is substantially reduced. This chapter introduces some of the key concepts of preparing patents. This chapter is by no means a substitute for your intellectual property attorney, but its contents will allow you to communicate more efficiently with your legal counsel.

RECORD OF INVENTION AND PRIORITY DATE

Timing is everything in patents. Although you might strive to be first to publish a manuscript, it is far more critical to beat the competition in the case of patents. A publication that is "scooped" is generally still cited in the literature and recognized as an important contribution. However, a patent that is "scooped" is a waste of money and effort; it is never issued and never rewarded.

The concept of timing differs throughout the world. In the United States, patents are awarded to the person who is "first to invent." In cases in which there is a conflict of priority (an automatic occurrence for two similar patent applications filed within 6 months of each other), a patent court uses laboratory records documenting the first evidence of the invention in order to reach a decision. In Europe and the majority of the World Trade Organization (WTO), priority is determined solely by who was the "first to file"; in other words, the "priority date" is everything.

The timing of invention (often called "reduction to practice") can be established in several ways in the United States. One is by the records established in bound laboratory notebooks that have been routinely signed, witnessed, and dated on a regular basis. Another is by a Record of Invention filed by the investigator/inventor within his or her own institution. This is a formal document prepared in conjunction with the Technology Transfer Office stating the idea that will be patented, the inventors of the idea, and the date. It is best to combine this with the signed and dated copies of notebook pages outlining the data contributing to the invention and the original statement of the invention, if this exists.

A safer way to protect the date of invention is to establish a "priority date," or filing date, by filing a Provisional Patent Application. This is a document that can be filed in the U.S. Patent and Trademark Office (USPTO) to establish the date of invention. It generally includes all of the data to be filed, a statement of the invention, and any background information (e.g., publications, patents) that may be required. There are no formal documentation requirements for a Provisional Patent Application since it is not actually examined by the patent office. However, it must adequately disclose the broadest aspects of the invention.

PATENTABILITY

What can be patented? The right to patent an idea or invention is established in the U.S. Constitution. The USPTO determines the merits of a patent application based on three criteria: novelty, utility, and nonobviousness. A novel idea must not have been known or used by anyone in the public domain (worldwide) prior to the patent application. Moreover, you or anyone else cannot have used the idea in a commercial manner for more than 1 year prior to the filing date. If your company has made a novel discovery and you have offered it for sale or to customers in the form of a service, you jeopardize your opportunity to protect the product with a patent. Utility must be demonstrated to the patent office in the form of an example or application. The nonobviousness of the invention will be determined by "those skilled in the art"; in other words, a hypothetical colleague with training similar to your own should not be able to reach the identical conclusion without your help. To find out about existing inventions or patents similar to your own in the patent literature, you can search public web sites maintained by the USPTO (http://www.uspto.gov) and the European Patent Office (EPO) (http://www.european-patent-office.org).

Patent Alternatives

When you have a novel idea, you have several options. One is to file a patent application. This will require significant investment of time and financial resources due to legal and filing fees. Alternatively, you can keep the information as a "trade secret." This will require significant diligence on the part of your company to maintain secrecy of the information, and it is particularly difficult in companies with employee turnover. Third, you can place the information into the public domain by publishing. This will discourage others from trying to patent the exact idea and make it possible for anyone to use the technology. However, it may inhibit business concerns from pursuing the technology since the absence of a patent will reduce the level of protection any company can place on future products.

Exclusivity

What does a patent do for you? A patent gives you the right to control the use of your idea. You can exclude others from making, using, or selling your invention. Before someone can "practice" your invention, they will need to obtain permission (a license) from you, the existing patent holder. Just as you can restrict everyone else's access to your ideas, others can do the same to you. If you ignore this restriction, you will "infringe" on an existing patent and open yourself to potential litigation and fines. It is far simpler to pay a flat rate (fee) or percentage of profits (royalty) to the patent assignee (owner) for a license to use his or her intellectual property.

There are strategic considerations in writing a patent. The precise legal language used can make the difference between a line on your curriculum vitae and a revenue-generating document. One of the most complex parts of the patent is the writing of the Claims, for which the exact choice of words has long-lasting consequences for the intellectual property. The subject of a claim may be a process (method), a machine or device, a manufactured article, or a composition of matter (a combination of a unique method and material); the latter has greatest value in the biotech arena. As a transitional phrase, the attorney may use "comprising" or "consisting of." "Comprising" means that the stated components of the claim may include other nonspecified elements, whereas "consisting of"

Table 6.1	*Components of a Patent*
Section	**Purpose**
Title of the Invention	Describe the invention.
Abstract	Briefly summarize the invention.
Background Information	What is the field of invention? What is the background of the related art?
Summary of Invention	What have you invented? This should be a description of the broadest aspect of your invention.
Description of Figures	Explain all accompanying figures.
Detailed Description of the Invention	Provide a description of the "preferred embodiment" of the invention and examples of its applications. Define critical terms or phrases.
Claims	Use single sentence phrases to define exactly what the patent "claims" as property. Components include a preamble (introducing the subject), a transitional phrase, and the body of the claim.

means that the specified components are the only ones that can be used. Claims may be "dependent" (referring back to earlier claims) or "independent" (standing alone). It is best to write your claims as broadly as possible so as not to restrict the area covered by your idea. Optimally, a patent should have a range of broad to narrow claims. It is recommended that you establish a sound working relationship with a good patent attorney; this will accelerate the filing and processing of strong patent applications and is worth the investment.

FILING

The filing process will require you to list all of the inventors on the application. This is defined as those people who actually came up with, or "conceived" of, the idea but not everyone who participated in the experiments. The filed patent application also can be "assigned" to someone or an organization. Most U.S. companies and universities require their scientists to sign over their rights to any intellectual property to their employers.

While the United States allows provisional patent filing, which is good for 1 year, most countries permit only a full or "nonprovisional" application for a patent. After filing a Nonprovisional Patent Application, you may revise the language of your claims to expand or restrict their content; however, you may not add "new matter" in the form of new data or background information. After reviewing the application, the patent examiner issues an "office action" in the form of a letter to the attorney and inventor outlining any restrictions or modifications that may be required. It is critical to remember that these office actions can be challenged and negotiated. Successful patent applicants receive a "notice of allowance" indicating that the patent will be issued upon receipt of the appropriate "issuing fee."

Patent offices around the world collect fees at various stages in the patent's life. A filing fee is required for each patent application. Rates vary from less than $1,000 to more than $10,000, depending on the country. Fees cover the process of translating the patent as well as the legal costs. Fees also are assessed when the patent is issued. During the interim, many foreign patent offices collect fees periodically (often yearly) to keep the patent application active. Following the issuance of a patent, many patent offices also charge "maintenance" fees assessed periodically during the life of the patent (20 years from the filing or priority date in the United States).

LICENSING

Now that you have just spent thousands of dollars in fees for legal services and patent applications, how do you realize gains from your patents? This occurs in the form of licenses and royalties. Technology transfer offices in universities attempt to license their patents to corporate entities. Their goals are to (1) immediately recover the costs of preparing and filing the patent application; (2) realize some tangible income in the form of upfront payments; (3) obtain additional future income in the form of payments at established milestones (preclinical outcomes, Phase I–III clinical trials, product launch); and (4) obtain royalty payments based on a percentage (anywhere from 2–6%) of gross sales of future products. In return, the industry will request that the university issue it an exclusive license to the technology and that it has the first right of refusal to any additional related intellectual property. Of course, the industry will negotiate for the lowest fees possible.

IMPLICATIONS FOR ACADEMIC AND INDUSTRY RELATIONS

The patent application process imposes some restrictions on the association between universities and companies. Both entities wish to retain their rights to the intellectual property resulting from joint research activities. Material transfer agreements (MTAs) and confidential disclosure agreements (CDAs) provide both parties with a mechanism to define the limits of their association and to mutually protect intellectual property. To protect their goals, companies may retain the services of university professors under consultancy agreements as compared to grants or sponsored research agreements. As consultants, the professors are able to provide intellectual contributions to the company outside their commitment to their academic employers. Likewise, universities protect their academic freedom by insisting on specific clauses in contracts that limit the company's ability to restrict publication of any data resulting from sponsored research agreements. In general, companies can hold up a publication describing sponsored research for only 30–90 days. This is sufficient time to allow for the filing of any patents or the modification of existing claims necessary to protect new intellectual property.

REFERENCE

Gordon, T. T., and Cookfair, A. S. *Patent Fundamentals for Scientists and Engineers*, 2nd ed. Boca Raton, FL: CRC Lewis Publishers, Inc., 1995.

7

·········

THE FEDERAL BIOLOGICS/DRUG/DEVICE APPROVAL PROCESS

················

The deans of medical schools and other university administrators see translational clinical research as an important academic goal. Likewise, in biotechnology, the intent of research is to support the development of a commercial clinical product. In the eyes of federal regulatory agencies, this can take the form of a drug, a device, or a biologic. This chapter introduces the general process of meeting regulatory standards in the development of a clinical product. Chapters 8–12 will expand on specific features of this process.

In the best of all possible worlds, your scientific research will lead to a product with clinical utility. This product may take the form of a therapeutic (drug, protein, nucleic acid, or cell-based biologic), a diagnostic, or a device. It is likely that the U.S. Food and Drug Administration (FDA) or its equivalent agency in other countries will regulate the final product, regardless of its form. Without the FDA's approval, you will not be able to license, market, or sell your product for use in the United States. Likewise, you will need to meet regulatory standards in the European Union to obtain approval, designated by a Conformité Européenne (CE) certification, to distribute your product. The International Organization for Standardization (the source of ISO 9000) also sets management quality standards for manufacturing concerns.

The FDA is composed of multiple centers, three of which play a major role in the developing biotech industry: the Center for Biologics Evaluation & Research (CBER), the Center for Devices & Radiological Health (CDRH), and the Center for Drug Evaluation & Research (CDER). It is advantageous to contact the FDA as you design your research plans and communicate with its representatives as early as possible. The FDA will convene and assign a review panel to your company's product. This will include FDA reviewers with expertise in basic science, clinical issues related to your field, and Chemistry, Manufacturing, and Controls (CMC). You are free to consult these panel members for guidance as you proceed with your product development. Anyone embarking on this pathway is advised strongly to consult with the FDA as early and as often as possible to avoid unexpected surprises later in the process.

Adult stem cell–based therapeutics will serve as an example to outline the stages in the product design process:

1. Research: This is the basic or bench science involved in the initial discovery phase of the project. Using a stem cell–based therapeutic as an example, this would be the *in vitro* demonstration that an adult stem cell has the capacity to differentiate along a specific lineage pathway into the cells of tissue X. The studies would be conducted in a reproducible and documented manner and would optimize the growth conditions necessary to ensure that a high percentage of the cells display differentiation-specific markers.

2. Development (preclinical): This is the expansion or scale-up phase of the project. The development stage includes the scale up in production of the differentiated adult stem cells and the demonstration of their therapeutic potential *in vivo*, using an animal model involving damage and repair of tissue X. The preclinical studies would be conducted using a statistically relevant number of both male and female animals at multiple time points. It may be necessary to conduct the work in both a small and large animal model; primates may need to serve as the large animal model in certain circumstances. Animals would be injected or implanted with increasing doses of the undifferentiated and/or differentiated adult stem cells in a therapeutic manner to heal a tissue X defect. Studies will determine the maximum number of cells that can be injected into a recipient animal. In addition, the preclinical studies will address manufacturing issues, including how the adult stem cells will be prepared, stored, shipped, and labeled. It will be important to identify and characterize the various products required in the manufacturing process and the vendors supplying these materials in anticipation of regulatory reviews later in the process. The results of the preclinical studies will need to be documented in a defined and validated manner

and will include evidence of equipment certification, assay procedures, and accuracy of standards employed in the study. Rather than conducting the preclinical animal studies "in house," it may be necessary to use a contract research facility with Good Laboratory Practice (GLP) expertise.

3. Investigational new drug (IND): Prior to initiating any human subject investigations with its potential product, the biotech company must submit an IND application for its adult stem cell product. The IND will include the following items for the FDA's review:

    a. CMC information that includes (1) quality assurance and quality control procedures, (2) source materials and raw materials used in manufacturing the product, (3) handling and stability of the final product, and (4) labeling information on the final product. This must include the clinical indications (and contra-indications) for the product, how it is to be stored, how it is to be used, and any potential adverse effects that should be monitored by the physician and patient.

    b. Preclinical study findings documenting the pharmacology of the product in animal models and its toxicological evaluation. Any existing information concerning the product's action in human subjects should be included.

    c. Clinical trial protocol. The company must present (1) a detailed outline of the clinical studies it will perform, (2) its commitment to performing the study with informed consent by the patient subjects, (3) the qualifications of the medical practitioners who will carry out the study, and (4) information concerning the Institutional Review Board that will approve or disapprove of the study design.

The company cannot initiate its clinical study until at least 30 days after its submission of the Biologics License Application (BLA) or IND application. During this period, the FDA can respond to the application by requesting additional information, documentation, or experiments. Alternatively, the FDA may deny approval of the product at this stage. If the company has not heard from the FDA at the end of the 30-day period, it may initiate its clinical trial.

4. Clinical trials (Phase I–III): This stage is the initial testing of the potential product in human subjects. The clinical trials will require coordination with physicians, patients, and hospitals as well as monitoring and oversight by both an Institutional Review Board (IRB) and in-house medical/clinical experts. It may be necessary to involve a "for-hire" Contract Research Organization (CRO) to provide some of these functions. Phase I studies focus almost exclusively on safety issues and involve only a small number of patients. The initial Phase I cohort of three to five patients would be exposed to 1/20th of the maximum

adult stem cell dose used in the preclinical studies. Based on the outcomes observed in these subjects, further cohorts would be exposed to cell doses increased by a factor of 0.33 or $\log_{10}1/2$; the absence of any adverse effects would need to be documented in each cohort before advancing the dose. Once the Phase I subjects had been monitored for a sufficient period of time, the study would advance to a limited Phase II analysis. Here, a larger number (10–40 subjects) would receive the cell product as a therapeutic. The clinical investigators would evaluate the product for both safety and efficacy. A control product, representing the current state of medical practice, may be used in parallel. Efficacy will need to be assessed relative to quantifiable benchmarks concerning the repair and recovery of function in tissue X. Successful outcomes in Phase II would be followed by a larger (50–250 subjects) Phase III analysis to obtain statistically significant data confirming the safety and efficacy of the therapeutic. The cost of a full-scale clinical trial exceeds the budget of many small biotech start-ups and may require a strategic partnership with a corporate sponsor. A biotech company may need to conduct multiple Phase I–III clinical trials in its development of a single product.

5. Biologics License Application (BLA): Upon completion of its clinical trials, the company may submit a BLA. This is required for any of the following products: autologous manipulated cells, blood or blood-derived materials, recombinant DNA plasmids or therapeutic recombinant DNA-derived products, monoclonal antibodies for use *in vivo*, and vaccines. The major sections included in the BLA (excluding the summary, cover letter, and table of contents) are outlined in Table 7.1. For a detailed description of the BLA document and its contents, refer to the FDA Guidance document at http://www.fda.gov/OHRMS/DOCKETS/98fr/980316g2.pdf. Since the FDA documents are revised frequently, you should search for updates or modifications of the BLA at the FDA web site (http://www.fda.gov).

The FDA can accept or reject the BLA for its review. If accepted for review, the FDA can take up to 1 year or more to reach its judgment. To meet the FDA's approval, your product must be examined and determined to meet the standards established in your BLA. In addition, it must be available for inspection throughout its manufacturing process and in its final form. If the FDA determines that any step in the manufacturing process will "impair the assurances of the continued safety, purity, and potency" of the product, it will not be approved. If your product passes inspection, the FDA will send your company a letter of approval that will list those sites that are authorized to manufacture the final product. The letter serves as the company's license to manufacture the product for interstate commerce.

Table 7.1   Major Sections Within the Biologics License Application

Labeling: How the product is labeled on the container, the package, and the package insert

Chemistry, Manufacturing, and Controls (CMC): Includes subsections on the biological substance, biological product, investigational formulation, environmental assessment, methods validation, batch records, and publications

Nonclinical Pharmacology and Toxicology: Includes subsections on pharmacology, pharmacokinetics, toxicology, data sets, and publications

Human Pharmacology and Bioavailability/Bioequivalence: Includes subsections with study reports on product bioavailability, bioequivalence, human biomaterials, human pharmacokinetics, and human pharmacodynamics as well as assays employed and any publications

Clinical Microbiology

Clinical Section: Includes subsections relating to the product's indications, safety, efficacy, and benefits/risks

Safety Update Report

Statistics

Case Report Tabulations: Includes the following patient subject information: demographics, inclusion/exclusion criteria, concomitant medications, medical histories, lab results (chemistry, hematology, urinalysis), efficacy, pharmacology/bioavailability/bioequivalence, and adverse events

Case Report Forms: Includes a copy of the case report form(s) used in the clinical studies

Patent Information

Patent Certifications

Establishment Certification: Includes information about the manufacturing establishment, including the water system, heat/ventilation and air conditioning (HVAC) systems, contamination and cross contamination, and lyophilization, as well as any diagrams of the structure and relevant publications

---

6. Postmarketing monitoring: Following the approval of a BLA or, in the case of a drug, a New Drug Application (NDA), the company has met the regulatory requirements necessary to market, license, and/or sell its product. Nevertheless, after this stage, it will be necessary to monitor the product users for any signs of adverse events. The company will be obligated to report these to the FDA in a timely manner. Depending on their severity, these may result in no changes in the product's use, the inclusion of a warning on the package insert to physicians and patients about the adverse event, or the withdrawal of the product from the market pending further testing and/or modifications.

Clearly, the product development process calls for more than simply scientific expertise. Chapters 8–12 will expand on some of the critical manufacturing and regulatory tools you will need for product development.

REFERENCES

http://www.oecd.org/about/0,2337,en_2649_34381_1_1_1_1_1,00.html Good Laboratory Practices (GLPs) in EU.

http://pharmacos.eudra.org/F2/eudralex/vol-1/home.htm Good Manufacturing Practices (GMPs) in EU.

http://www.fda.gov/cber/ Web site for the Center for Biologics Evaluation and Research (CBER).

http://www.fda.gov/cdrh/ Web site for the Center for Devices and Radiological Health (CDRH).

http://www.fda.gov/cder/ Web site for the Center for Drug Evaluation and Research (CDER).

http://www.emea.eu.int/ Web site for the European Agency for the Evaluation of Medicinal Products (EMEA).

http://www.iso.ch/iso/en/ISOOnline.openerpage Web site for the International Organization for Standardization (ISO).

http://www.fda.gov/cder/regulatory/applications/ind_page_1.htm Web site for Investigational New Drug (IND) applications.

http://www.fda.gov/cber/minutes/351bio.htm Web site recording the initial implementation of the Biologics License process.

http://www.fda.gov/ Web site for the U.S. Food and Drug Administration (FDA).

http://www.cenorm.be/ European Committee for Standardization.

chapter

8

· · · · · · · · · ·

GOOD LABORATORY PRACTICES AND CURRENT GOOD MANUFACTURING PRACTICES

· · · · · · · · · · · · · · · · ·

Document tracking and the maintenance of detailed records are critical components throughout all steps of the discovery, development, and manufacturing process. Nevertheless, despite the fact that scientific training focuses extensively on the role of record keeping in its day-to-day operation, academic scientists traditionally have a hard time embracing and integrating basic manufacturing concepts into their repertoire. This reflects a difference in culture. Manufacturing seeks to achieve absolute reproducibility in its process; any deviation is seen as a failure. In contrast, basic research thrives on novelty, innovation, and the serendipitous finding; thus, deviation from standard protocol is the norm. This chapter covers one of the most important topics in biotechnology: the interface with federal manufacturing regulations.

DEFINITIONS OF GLP AND cGMP

The Code of Federal Regulations (21) contains guidelines for defining Good Laboratory Practices (GLP) and current Good Manufacturing Practices

45

(cGMP). The U.S. Food and Drug Administration (FDA) has developed these rules to ensure that accepted scientific and manufacturing practices are used in preclinical laboratory research supporting product safety (GLP) and in the manufacture, labeling, and distribution of safe and effective products (cGMP).

Several themes underlie all aspects of these regulations. First and foremost is **documentation** at all levels of the process. The records must include certain key information, such as the names of individuals with the **authorization** and **responsibility** to oversee the conduct of a study or process. Ultimately, these individuals are **accountable** for the results and conclusions of any experiments and reports. **Standardized** documents provide a system to ensure the **reproducibility** of any experimental protocol or manufacturing process and the **traceability** of the various reagents, solutions, and components used. Ultimately, the records provide a history and **verification** mechanism for audits by internal or external inspectors, although onsite observation is also required.

All the documents in the world are useless if you have no way to access them. It is critical to establish a document control system. Someone in the laboratory or organization must be responsible for organizing and maintaining the files of the documents and records. You need to keep all official versions of a document on file in a biotech company. Eventually, these will have regulatory importance. You need to factor this time-consuming and demanding job into your plans while building your laboratory from the ground up. Make sure you allocate the necessary personnel resources to this task early on. It will reduce the effort and disorganization/reorganization required to implement the same measures at a later date after your personnel and staff have developed their own habits and data control procedures.

Table 8.1   The –tion and -ility Issues
Authorization
Certification
Documentation
Standardization
Validation
Verification
Accountability
Reproducibility
Responsibility
Traceability

The documents themselves include some common features. Each document needs to define who is responsible for establishing the procedure, supervising it, and actually carrying it out. The authorizing officials must sign and date the original documents; copies can later be distributed to staff personnel in hard copy or electronic format. The document should include a statement describing its purpose (i.e., what the procedure is for). Generally, documents also include sections identifying any related or supporting documents as well as any references pertinent to its contents.

Documents for specific tasks should include some means to verify that the operator is actually complying with the stated protocol. For example, a particular step in the protocol will include a specific section that the operator initials and dates (with the time). In manufacturing procedures, a member of the Quality Assurance Unit (QAU) may also witness this section with his or her signature. Alternatively, there may be a log sheet associated with a piece of equipment that is signed and dated whenever a maintenance procedure is carried out.

Documents and records establish the routine operation of the laboratory and the manufacturing process. They serve an equally important purpose by recording any incidents or deviations from this routine. Protocols and procedures need to be established to deal with (1) personal injuries or accidents that occur to an operator during a procedure, (2) any unauthorized deviations from accepted experimental or manufacturing protocols, (3) contamination of cell or tissue cultures, and (4) unanticipated animal illness or death during an experiment. Additional procedures for unexpected incidents may be required depending on the nature of your experiments.

Document procedures need to be established for all steps in a research program and/or manufacturing process. Academic scientists may see these steps as unnecessary in early, discovery-stage research, but this view is shortsighted. With proper planning, you can embed a structure within your document procedures that automatically collects and collates all of the data you will need for future analyses. This can be applied to experimental design processes, discovery research, and development and manufacturing issues. The existence of these documents will simplify the final review and ultimate regulatory approval of any resulting products. In addition, they will make it easier for you to outline, write, and publish manuscripts describing your findings in peer-reviewed journals.

DOCUMENTATION PROCEDURES

There are many types of documents. **Descriptive** documents instruct how a process or procedure is done, documents focused on **data collection**

Table 8.2 Document Types (from http://www.biotech.nhctc.edu)	
Types of Documents	*Examples*
Descriptive	Standard operating procedures (SOPs)
	Protocols
	Master production records
Data collection	Forms
	Reports
	Production batch records
	Log books
Numbering systems	Part number
	Lot number
	Equipment number
	Form number
	SOP number
	Report number
Data files	Equipment history files
	Facility qualification files
	Product files
	Experimental report files
Notebooks	Laboratory

provide forms or reports for raw data in experiments or manufacturing, and **numbering systems** documents provide a standardized method for identifying and labeling records in the discovery, development, and manufacturing process. In addition, **data files** provide a mechanism for systematically archiving and storing records related to equipment, facilities' qualifications, and products, and the majority of a laboratory's raw data is traditionally recorded in **notebooks**. All of these document types share the intent to ensure reproducibility and accountability within a process.

Each laboratory needs to establish clear and straightforward written procedures defining how to conduct routine operations. These operations include, but are not limited to, the following:

- Experimental protocols
- Equipment maintenance
- Equipment repair
- Media and solution preparation
- Tissue culture and cell isolation
- Animal procedures
- Safety procedures

- Cleaning procedures
- Biohazard and chemical waste disposal
- Radioisotope usage
- Labeling procedures for materials or products
- Mechanisms to deal with deviations from established protocols

VALIDATION PROTOCOLS

In addition to documenting procedures, you must also document the equipment used. Each piece of equipment must be validated with respect to its **installation, operation**, and **performance qualifications**. A licensed testing company must evaluate the equipment with known standards and periodically certify it to ensure its continued accuracy.

The Validation Protocols listed in Table 8.3 make up a data collection document. The questions each qualification process needs to address are presented in the next subsection.

Installation Qualifications

1. Equipment identification information: What are the manufacturer's model and serial number, size, dimension, capacity, and location?
2. Equipment utility requirements: Does it need water, gas, electric, compressed air, steam, drain, or liquid nitrogen? What are the specific dimensions, operating capacities, or parameters of any of these needs?
3. Equipment safety features: Does the equipment have alarms, settings to activate the alarms, or pressure relief valves?

Operational Qualifications

1. Equipment calibration requirements: What parameters need to be measured? How will measurement be accomplished? What are the acceptable ranges or limits for these parameters?

Table 8.3   Validation Protocols (from http://www.biotech.nhctc.edu)
Installation Qualification (IQ)
Operational Qualification (OQ)
Performance Qualification (PQ)

2. Preoperational requirements: Does the equipment need to be cleaned or sterilized? Does the computer software need to be installed?
3. Operational criteria: How do you actually run the equipment? What constitutes an acceptable performance?
4. Validation acceptance criteria: What defines the specific parameters that need to be met for validation?

Performance Qualifications

1. Preliminary operations: Does the equipment meet the validation acceptance criteria while you are testing minimum and maximum processing conditions (i.e., while you are establishing the limits of its operation)?
2. Performance qualification procedures: Does the equipment successfully meet the validation acceptance criteria during three consecutive cycles?
3. Performance qualification acceptance criteria: Can you document that the equipment met all of the validation acceptance criteria parameters? Do you have the raw data and number of consecutive runs to meet this requirement?

INVENTORIES

It is simplest to organize an inventory to maintain a record of the physical resources within your laboratory. You will greatly reduce the work involved if you establish these inventories as you first set up the laboratory. The major inventory areas and subcategories to consider are listed below.
1. Antibodies
   a. Source (manufacturer or provider)
   b. Catalog number
   c. Monoclonal (specie) or polyclonal (specie)
   d. Immunoglobulin type
   e. Antigen (specie of origin)
   f. Recommended titer for immunoblot, immunoprecipitation, histology
   g. Storage temperature and location
   h. References
   i. Date
   j. Operator name
2. Biologicals
   a. Tissue type
   b. Specie and characterization (age, gender, height, weight, ethnicity)

   c. Source (referring physician)

   d. Processing procedure (formalin fixed, flash frozen, paraffin embedded, etc.)

   e. Storage temperature and location

   f. Date

   g. Operator name

3. Cells

   a. Cell type

   b. Specie and tissue of origin

   c. Primary culture, clone, or cell line

   d. Source (American Type Culture Collection catalog number or other identification)

   e. Cell concentration (cells/ml and/or cells/vial)

   f. Storage temperature and location

   g. References

   h. Date

   i. Operator name

4. Consumables

   a. Type

   b. Source (manufacturer name and catalog number)

   c. Receipt date

   d. Storage location

   e. Operator identification

5. Chemicals

   a. Chemical name

   b. Chemical formula

   c. Molecular weight

   d. Chemical Abstracts Services (CAS) reference number

   e. Source (manufacturer name and catalog number)

   f. Material Safety Data Sheet link

   g. Storage temperature and location

   h. Date

   i. Operator name

6. Equipment

   a. Type

   b. Manufacturer name, model number, and serial number

   c. Receipt date

   d. Cost

   e. Installation qualification date

   f. Operational qualification date

   g. Performance qualification date

   h. Maintenance records (dates, operator identification)

   i. Certification records (dates, operator identification)

    j. Utilization records

    k. Date for next scheduled maintenance

    l. Data entry operator identification

7. Plasmids

    a. Vector type and size

    b. cDNA insert (specie of origin, size, gene identifier)

    c. Source of plasmid (manufacturer name, catalog number, or name of academic investigator including address, phone, and e-mail contact information)

    d. References

    e. Physical state (glycerol stock, aqueous, ethanol, lyophilized)

    f. Storage temperature and location

    g. Date of preparation

    h. Utilization dates

    i. Data entry operator identification

8. Oligonucleotides

    a. Source (manufacturer)

    b. Identification of DNA (gene name, specie, Genbank ID number)

    c. Base pair sequence

    d. Melting temperature

    e. Polymerase Chain Reaction (PCR) cycle conditions (if relevant)

    f. Physical state (glycerol stock, aqueous, ethanol, lyophilized)

    g. Storage temperature and location

    h. Date of preparation

    i. Utilization dates

    j. Data entry operator identification

9. Notebooks

    a. Inventory control number assigned to notebook

    b. Date of issue

    c. Date of return

    d. To whom notebook was issued

    e. Who issued notebook

    f. Who received notebook upon return

    g. Certification that the notebook pages are signed and witnessed

    h. Storage location of notebook

    i. Data entry operator identification and date

NOTEBOOKS

In a research and discovery laboratory, the laboratory notebook is the fundamental method for recording raw data. In keeping your notebooks, you need to resurrect the practices you learned (or resisted) in freshman quantitative analytical chemistry. The notebook provides a contemporaneous scientific record; you record observations as you make them. You need to use a bound rather than loose-leaf notebook to assure future auditors that the data entry occurred sequentially rather than piecemeal. You need to use indelible ink to make your entries. This will reduce the risk that your data will dissolve if you have the misfortune to spill a Coke or other aqueous or ethanol-based liquid solvent on your notebook (outside the laboratory, of course!). You should make a habit of recording your experimental design, your raw data and observations, and your ideas in a legible and orderly format. Because your notebook is also a legal document, you should sign each page and date it upon completion. If you tape another printed page into your notebook, you should sign it so that your signature and the date overlap both the insert and the actual page of the notebook. A fellow employee should witness each page of your notebook. Preferably, this will be someone who is not directly involved in the project but is knowledgeable in your field (i.e., he or she should be able to understand the contents of the notebook).

All of these steps have important patent implications. In the European Union and much of the world, patents are awarded to the first inventor to file an application. In the United States, patents are awarded to the applicant who is determined to be the first to invent. In the event that your patent application faces an interference from a pending or issued patent, you will discover that careful notebook records can save (or lose) your day in court. If kept correctly, your notebook may determine that you, rather than a competing organization, made the first observations relating to the patent.

FEDERAL REGULATIONS

The regulations pertaining to biotech continue to undergo review and revision by the U.S. Food and Drug Administration (FDA) and other federal agencies. For specific procedures or products, you are advised to contact the FDA or relevant regulatory agency for guidance. You cannot incorporate quality assurance procedures too soon if you are serious about your commercial development strategy. New companies should seek out manufacturing and quality assurance expertise at the time of their incorporation, if not earlier. This expert should have some prior experience working with the FDA, preferably with the branch that will most likely oversee your particular product. You will increase your likelihood of success by directly approaching the FDA and letting its input guide the growth and direction of your company's future.

In some respects, GLP and cGMP are abstract concepts, particularly if you have never had industrial experience; however, they have very concrete consequences. Remember that these are federal regulations. If your laboratory fails to comply with them, you may face legal challenges. In addition to fines and restrictions on the sale of your products, you could face the threat of criminal charges and imprisonment. The intent of GLP and cGMP is to ensure that the public receives safe and effective products from manufacturers. Even if you do not fully appreciate the nuances underlying a particular mandate of the law, it is in your interest (and your company's) to find a way to incorporate it into your laboratory's operation and your company's culture. After all, you do not have to be a highway engineer to understand why they post speeding regulations.

INSPECTION PROCESS

To give you some idea of the complexity and detail expected of GLP operations, the following table and sections catalog the type of questions that FDA inspectors will ask when evaluating a nonclinical laboratory safety study to ensure compliance. The cGMP process involves even greater scrutiny and focuses on and monitors additional features, such as product packaging.

Components of a GLP Inspection/Audit

Organization and Personnel

- What does the organization chart of the laboratory look like?
- Who is the study director?
- What are his or her qualifications and expertise?

Table 8.4   Components of a GLP Inspection/Audit (from http://www.fda.gov/ora/compliance_ref/bimo/7348_808/part_III.html)
Organization and Personnel
Quality Assurance Unit (QAU)
Facilities
Equipment
Testing Facilities Operations
Reagents and Solutions
Animal Care
Test and Control Article Specifications
Protocol and Conduct of Nonclinical Laboratory Studies
Records and Reports

- How is the study director selected and, if necessary, replaced?
- How is information transmitted between the study director, Quality Assurance Unit (QAU), laboratory personnel, and study sponsors?
- How is the computerization of the study established, validated, and operated?

Quality Assurance Unit (QAU)

- Do standard operating procedures (SOPs) exist for all steps in the experiment or process?
- Have records of all changes and amendments to the SOPs been maintained?
- Has a master schedule of all the experiments or processes been maintained?
- Does the QAU inspect the preclinical laboratory studies to ensure their integrity?
- How are in-process inspections scheduled and audited?
- Does the QAU notify the study director if problems are detected in the study's integrity?
- How rapidly does notification occur?
- Does the QAU submit status reports to the study director?
- Does the QAU review the final reports of the study?

Facilities

- What is the floor plan of the facility?
- Are there environmental controls and monitoring procedures for critical areas?
- Does the laboratory have SOPs listing the materials and methods for cleaning the facility?
- Are there specific areas identified for the receipt, storage, mixing, and handling of control and test articles?
- Are specific functions within the laboratory performed in separate rooms?
- Are archived records and computers protected from temperature, water, or electromagnetic damage?
- Are there temperature and humidity records for the facility?

Equipment

- Is the equipment suitable to support the generation of valid results?
- Is the equipment clean and easy to use?

- Where is it located?
- Are the air conditioning, heating, and ventilation systems sufficient to support the operation of the equipment?
- Is the equipment dedicated to a particular use?
- Is the nondedicated equipment decontaminated prior to the preparation of a test or control article?
- Do all of the critical pieces of equipment have the following documents: SOP, operations manual, maintenance schedule and log record, calibration/standardization procedure, schedule, and log?

Testing Facilities Operations

- Does the laboratory have established SOPs for all aspects of its operation? If so, does it actually follow its SOPs?
- Are the SOPs kept up-to-date?
- Have the SOPs been reviewed and authorized by the appropriate responsible personnel or managers?
- Is there an historical file record of all changes and amendments to the SOPs?
- How are personnel trained on a particular SOP?
- How do they perform a particular SOP?
- Do the personnel adhere to the SOP?

Reagents and Solutions

- What is the quality of the laboratory's reagents and solutions?
- How does the laboratory go about purchasing, receiving, labeling, and determining the acceptability of its reagents and solutions?
- Are these procedures followed?

Animal Care

- Are the laboratory's animals housed in a way that will not influence the study's outcome?
- Do SOPs exist concerning the environment, housing, feeding, handling, and care of the laboratory animals? Are they followed?
- Are there pest control procedures?
- Does the laboratory have an Institutional Animal Care and Use Committee (IACUC)? If so, does it have SOPs defining and minutes recording its operation? Do the identification tags on the animals match the identity cards on their cages?
- Are water and food samples analyzed for purity and content?
- Are records maintained of these analyses?
- Are animals of different species housed in separate rooms?

Test and Control Article Specifications

- How does the laboratory acquire, receive, and store its control and test articles to prevent contamination and deterioration?
- How are the purity, composition, and/or strength of the control and test articles defined?
- Are control and test articles retained for all studies extending for more than 4 weeks?
- How are mixtures of control or test articles prepared?
- Are the mixtures uniform?

Protocol and Conduct of Nonclinical Laboratory Studies

- Are the study protocol and its supporting SOPs written and authorized appropriately?
- Can it be verified that the protocol and SOPs are followed?
- How are the test systems monitored?
- How is the raw data recorded?
- How are corrections to the raw data made (do they obscure the original data; are they initialed, dated, and explained by the operator)?
- How is the test system randomized?
- How are specimens collected and identified?
- Who has the authority to access the data and archival and computer records?

Records and Reports

- How does the laboratory store and retrieve documents and records?
- Are records (i.e., raw data, documents, protocols, amendments, revisions, final reports, specimens) retained? For how long? Are they indexed for easy retrieval? Are they stored in an environmentally controlled space to prevent deterioration? Can the records be transferred to an electronic format within the laboratory?
- Are the raw data original, accurate, legible, attributable to the original observer, and recorded at the actual time of observation?
- Do the protocol and its SOPs match the final report?
- Does the final report match the raw data?
- Do the interim reports conform to the final report?
- Do the retained specimens conform to the final report?
- For animal studies, confirm that the following records can be traced:
  - Animal body weights
  - Food and water consumption
  - Test system observation and dosing

- Analysis of uniformity, concentration, and stability of the test and control articles
- Protocols for analyses (clinical chemistry, hematology, urinalyses)
- Necropsy and gross pathology
- Histopathology

REFERENCES

http://www.access.gpo.gov/nara/cfr/waisidx_99/21cfr600_99.html Biological products information from Department of Health and Human Services.

http://www.fda.gov/cder/dmpq/cgmpregs.htm Center for Drug Evaluation and Research (CDER), Code of Federal Regulations, Current Good Manufacturing Practices (cGMPs).

http://www.fda.gov/cder/guidance/index.htm CDER Guidance Documents.

http://www.bio-link.org/GMPtoc.htm Good Manufacturing Practices (GMPs) information from Bio-Link.

http://www.access.gpo.gov/cgi-bin/cfrassemble.cgi?title=199921 National Archives and Records Administration's Code of Federal Regulations.

http://www.fda.gov/ora/compliance_ref/bimo/7348_808/part_III.html Office of Regulatory Affairs (ORA) compliance inspections information.

http://www.biotech.nhctc.edu Introductory material for BT220: Biotechnology Manufacturing.

chapter

9

· · · · · · · · · ·

EXPERIMENTAL PROTOCOLS

· · · · · · · · · · · · · · · · ·

Research plays a seminal role in the product development pipeline. Through research, scientists discover the ideas that eventually will lead to a commercial clinical application. Regulatory agencies want to know how this takes place in both academia and biotechnology. Industry has developed a series of standardized documents to capture the steps in this process. The process of developing these documents has utility for scientists in both academia and biotech. This chapter focuses on the initial document in the chain: the experimental protocol (also known as a test protocol).

PROACTIVE DESIGN AND TROUBLESHOOTING: LESSONS FROM ENGINEERS

One of the lures of a scientific career is the chance to chart out new territory and to reveal previously unknown ideas. It almost seems heretical to suggest that the "discovery" process of science can be organized and standardized. Nevertheless, the two concepts are compatible. The engineering community has refined the art of problem solving into a well-defined process. This same approach can be applied to biological questions.

Organization and Content

An essential component of the process of designing an experimental protocol is to commit your ideas to paper in an organized manner, thereby

59

providing yourself and your colleagues with a record of how the project evolved (See Table 9.1). Before conducting an experiment, the first step is to define your **objective**. Craft the hypothetical question that you are setting out to answer in its simplest form. In the final analysis, you should be able to provide it with a "yes" or "no" answer.

The second step is to identify the **background** information critical to the issue. Although you may be fully aware of the scientific literature relating to the question, assume that anyone who reads your document has no such knowledge. You need to provide a concise outline identifying the key facts that are relevant to your hypothesis. You should refer to a list of **references** that are essential to your argument. This list should include references with data both supporting and refuting your hypothesis, if they exist.

Your experiment will undoubtedly require the use of your time, resources, and energy. You will need to convince the skeptic that there is an underlying **rationale** that makes this use of resources worthwhile. Your rationale needs to address several levels of concern:

- How will it benefit society (i.e., will you cure a medical disease)?
- How will it benefit your institution (i.e., will you generate data for a grant, manuscript, or patent)?
- How will it benefit you (i.e., will it allow you to meet your personal objective of a thesis, job offer, or promotion)?

The third step in designing an experimental protocol is to reduce the concept to practice. This involves detailed planning and organization. You need to identify all of the **equipment and materials** you will need. Your lists should include the name of each piece of equipment or supply, the manufacturer or vendor and its contact information, and either the model number or catalog number.

In addition, you need to outline the steps in the **experimental procedure**. Do not make the mistake of omitting various steps because they appear obvious to you; include everything. If you and your staff perform a

Table 9.1 Experimental Protocol	
Objective	What question are you asking?
Background and Rationale	Why should you ask it?
References	What is relevant to the question?
Equipment and Materials	What tools do you need?
Experimental Procedures	What will you actually do?
Outcome Criteria	What should you expect to happen?

procedure daily, you may assume that everyone completes it accurately even though this is often not the case. Each individual may perform specific steps in a different order or with slightly different reagents. Such variation in technique can lead to inconsistent results and experimental error. In addition, staff turnover is a fact of life in both academic and biotech laboratories. Even if your current staff is performing the procedure consistently, a well-written experimental procedure will allow you to rapidly and reproducibly train any new personnel you hire. When documenting your procedure, make a concerted effort to identify both the positive and negative controls you will include in the study. The information in these sections serves several purposes: (1) it quickly allows you to calculate the cost of the project, (2) it provides you with the chance to anticipate any problems or shortcomings in the experimental design, and (3) it provides a document that presents your ideas to colleagues or supervisors for their critique.

The fourth, and final, step in designing an experimental protocol is to list the **outcome criteria** you anticipate from the study. Even before you collect the data, you should have a clear idea of what results you expect. Specifically, you know how the positive and negative of controls should behave. If either of these controls fails, the experiment is not acceptable. Likewise, you should have some expectation of how the experimental outcome will behave relative to the controls. For example, if you are assaying for the presence of an inducing factor, you can define the percentage or fold stimulation above background levels that will constitute the presence of a "true" inducing factor. If possible, use statistical methods to reach these values; you may rely on the data from similar experiments conducted in your own laboratory or from the literature to perform such calculations. This statistical analysis will allow you to determine how many times you may need to repeat the study. You will need to run many more replicates of the assay if you are searching for a 20% change versus a 20-fold change in the outcome. By identifying these values objectively in advance, you will have reduced the level of subjectivity in your interpretation of the final experimental results.

10

· · · · · · · · · ·

EXPERIMENTAL REPORTS

· · · · · · · · · · · · · · · · ·

After you have conducted your initial experiment, you need to reduce the data into a coherent report. This takes time and effort on the part of the investigator and is not necessarily a routine step in academic laboratories. In contrast, biotechnology and industry view this as a critical element in their chain of discovery. This chapter discusses the composition of experimental reports (also known as test reports).

JUST THE FACTS, PLEASE!

In academia, an experimental endpoint is usually marked by a publication. The data are scattered across multiple records within notebooks and computer files. In biotech, you need to capture and collage your data in transit. The experimental report provides an organized and reproducible format to accomplish this. It is designed to complement the format of the experimental protocol. This process serves three major needs: (1) it concisely reports the factual outcomes of the experiment; (2) it places these facts in direct juxtaposition with the study's conclusions, allowing readers to determine for themselves whether the data support the conclusions, and (3) the process creates a single document summarizing a body of work, allowing the information to be tracked and reported easily in the future.

Table 10.1 *Experimental Report Contents*	
Objective	***What did you originally set out to do?***
Experimental Results	What did you find out?
Exceptional Conditions/ Deviations	Did your experimental protocol differ from the original design? If so, how and why?
Discussion/Conclusions	Did your experiment meet your outcome criteria expectations? If not, why not?
Speculation	Did you discover something unexpected? Do you have any ideas for future experiments?

ORGANIZATION AND CONTENT

The **objective** should match that defined originally in the experimental protocol. It needs to reduce the hypothesis underlying your study to a single question that can be answered in either a "yes" or "no" manner.

The **experimental results** should define the study's outcome. The data needs to be presented in a concise manner. This can take a tabular form or include appendices with graphics of the data. It is highly recommended that the section include a statistical quantification of the results. Identify the number of times an experiment was conducted, the mean +/- standard deviation of the value, and the probability of its significance. If there is insufficient data to support a statistical analysis, state this fact. It is just as important to consider what the experimental results do *not* contain: conclusions, speculation, and interpretation. These belong in separate sections.

The best of all plans is subject to change. This can occur due to technical reasons, accidents, or the subsequent identification of an unexpected problem or barrier. Whenever there is a change in plan, this should be noted as an **exceptional condition or a deviation**. Include a description of the original plan, how you changed it, whether or not the change was performed in all replicates of the study, and an explanation of why the change occurred. This information will be critical to any future attempts to repeat your study, either by yourself or by others.

Once you have collected and tabulated your results, you are in a position to evaluate them in the context of your outcome criteria. In the **Discussion/Conclusions** section, you should systematically state whether your experiment satisfied each of the original outcome criteria. This section should concisely capture the conclusions supported by your data. If you believe your data supports conclusions in addition to those you originally identified in the experimental protocol, this is the place to state them. In addition, you should discuss your findings in the context of the existing literature. State whether your findings are in agreement or disagreement with others in the field.

The experimental report provides an opportunity to evaluate the experimental process in a go/no-go manner. In some ways, it is more difficult to stop something than it is to initiate it. In the **Speculation** section, you may need to address the following questions: Does your study suggest that further experiments in this area are not warranted? If so, why?

Hopefully, you will not need to take this negative approach. Instead, after doing all of the hard work, you will have come to the fun part. In the **Speculation** section, you have the opportunity to interpret your findings. If you can, address the following questions: Is there anything novel you can infer or extrapolate from your data? Does your study point to a logical set of future experiments?

In biotech, the experimental report serves as a record of the discovery process. In academia, it can serve as an interim step in the process of manuscript preparation. The extra effort you take to organize your data as you collect them and to commit your thoughts to paper will pay off. This approach will reduce the time you need to complete and publish your studies; try it!

11

· · · · · · · · · ·

EXPERIMENTAL METHODS

· · · · · · · · · · · · · · · ·

After you have conducted an experiment multiple times and confirmed the validity of your experimental protocol, it is time to promote the process to your institutional archives. This is accomplished by elevating the process to the status of an experimental method (also known as a test method). By doing so, you create a codified document that anyone in your laboratory can use with confidence of a successful outcome. You can also share the experimental method with other investigators who wish to reproduce your work in their own laboratories.

DETAILS OF ACCEPTED PRACTICE

When an experimental protocol has met the tests of time, it can be reduced to an experimental method. How do you know when this has occurred? If you are still modifying the method every other time you use it, it is probably too early. If you are ready to share the method with a colleague, you have definitely arrived at the necessary point. If you have completed the study so many times that you no longer feel compelled to record its details in your notebook, you have probably gone past the appropriate time point. Your job is to reduce the details of the accepted practice to a format that anyone could follow successfully, including your PhD thesis advisor! Theoretically, anyone should be able to pick up the document and conduct the method without direct supervision by you or anyone else. Table 11.1 outlines a process by which to accomplish this task.

Organization and Content

For the **Objective/Scope**, identify what the method accomplishes in its broadest sense. The scope of your experimental method can vary significantly. For example, if you are writing a method for performing an enzyme linked immunoabsorbent assay (ELISA), the purpose is to measure the concentration of protein or chemical using an antibody-based system. You will write the details of this method in a broad sense. Alternatively, if you are writing a method for measuring leptin using an ELISA, the scope of your method will be limited to a particular protein. In this case, the details of the method will be more specific.

In the **Responsibility** section, you need to identify whom to contact in the laboratory for back-up instruction pertaining to the method. For example, your ELISA method requires the use of a spectrophotometric plate reader. Since equipment is expensive to repair and replace, you do not want someone who does not know how to operate the plate reader attempting to conduct the experimental method unsupervised. The **Responsibility** section of the ELISA experimental method will instruct the reader to contact you (or someone else) for instruction in the use of this machine. To prevent the document from becoming dated as soon as you leave the laboratory, it is best to identify individuals based on their role in the laboratory (e.g., laboratory manager, senior research technician, senior postdoctoral fellow) rather than by name.

In the **References** section, you should list those documents that provided you with instruction in the method. These may include primary literature for methods you have developed *de novo*. For methods that are somewhat routine in the literature, you are encouraged to reference commercially available protocol manuals such as *Current Protocols in Molecular Biology* (http://www.interscience.wiley.com/). You may wonder why you should develop your own experimental method if detailed protocols already exist and have been compiled in great books like the

Table 11.1 *Experimental Method*	
Objective/Scope	What is the general purpose of the method?
	What is the specific purpose of the method?
Responsibility	Who should carry out the parts of the method?
References	Where should you look for additional information or background?
Materials and Equipment	What do you need to do the job?
Procedure	How do you do the job?
Appendix	Is there anything that will help make the job easier?

Current Protocols series. Despite the similarities in equipment and reagents, each laboratory is a unique environment. No matter how detailed a published method might be, you may discover that it lacks a few details specific to your own laboratory. In addition, no matter how well a method may work for the authors of a manual, you may need to introduce at least one "deviation" from that protocol to customize its use in your own laboratory. This can be due to differences in equipment, to innovations or products that post-date the publication of the textbook, or just to the fact that you like to be creative when you follow a recipe. The **References** section should also point the reader to any other experimental methods supporting documents within the laboratory that provide instruction in preparing reagents or performing individual substeps.

In the **Materials and Equipment** section, you should identify the essential items that the method calls for. This section should include the name of each item, its supplier or vendor, a catalog or model number, and the concentration of any required stock solutions. This section will make it much simpler for a novice to plan and prepare for the experimental method.

For the **Procedure**, write out a detailed list of each step in the experimental method. If you do this correctly, you will feel an excruciating, mind-numbing sensation throughout the process. This is normal. There is nothing too trivial that you can include. You will be doing future generations of laboratory personnel a favor by identifying which hand you hold your pipet in, how you open or close a tube single-handedly, and what volume of bleach you add to a container of waste media. Do not assume that it is demeaning to anyone else to provide this level of detail. Instead, people who use the experimental method with a different laboratory background than your own will gain the benefit of your experience!

Finally, in the **Appendix**, provide templates of tables, data collection forms, or checklists that you have developed for the experimental method. For example, you may have developed tried and true documents for collating absorbance data from 96 well plates in ELISA assays. This may be a hard-copy form that you paste into your notebook or a computer file that converts the absorbance data directly into antigen concentrations. Both of these accessory documents would be tremendous time-savers for future generations of research personnel. If you leave them a complete experimental method, they will be more likely to fondly remember your name long after you have moved on to new horizons.

REFERENCES

Ausubel, F. M., Brent, R., Kingston, R. E., Moore, D. D., Seidman, J. G., Smith, J. A., and Struhl, K. *Current Protocols in Molecular Biology* (4 volumes). Edison, NJ: John Wiley & Sons, 2004.

Bierer, B., Coligan, J. E., Margulies, D. H., Shevach, E. M., and Strober, W. *Current Protocols in Immunology* (4 volumes). Edison, NJ: John Wiley & Sons, 2004.

Bonifacino, J. S., Dasso, M., Harford, J. B., Lippincott-Schwartz, J., and Yamada, K. M. *Current Protocols in Cell Biology* (2 volumes). Edison, NJ: John Wiley & Sons, 2004.

Coligan, J. E., Dunn, B. M., Ploegh, H. L., Speicher, D. W., and Wingfield, P. T. *Current Protocols in Protein Science* (2 volumes). Edison, NJ: John Wiley & Sons, 2004.

12

··········

STANDARD OPERATING PROCEDURES

·················

The document trail in discovery research culminates in the standard operating procedure (SOP). This is the finalized version of how to do the job. This chapter briefly describes how the SOP goes one step beyond the experimental method.

What makes an SOP different from an experimental method? In a nutshell, the answer is rigidity. An experimental method is a well-defined, working document that *suggests* to an operator how a particular experiment *may* be conducted. In contrast, an SOP *instructs* an operator how a particular assay *must* be conducted.

While the operator has some latitude for change in an experimental method, he or she has none in an SOP. Essentially, an SOP is an experimental method that has been cast in concrete. It is something that works so well that it must not and cannot be changed (at least not without a major action within the Research and Development structure of the biotechnology company).

SOPs are important for two major reasons: they ensure reproducibility, and they generate documents that are suitable for an independent, external audit of operating procedures. For example, if your laboratory developed an assay that is used for the clinical diagnosis of a rare genetic disorder, you would want to minimize the possibility of false-positive or false-negative outcomes. If each operator conducts the same assay with minor variations, the chances of a false-positive or false-negative outcome are increased. Thus, reproducibility is a critical objective. Likewise, if the U.S. Food and Drug Administration (FDA) receives a complaint about your clinical diagnostic product and decides to audit your operation, you will want to have a system in place documenting how your personnel have been conducting the assay. Consequently, the best approach is to establish an SOP for the procedure.

There are several ways to ensure that the operator follows the SOP. One approach is to provide the SOP in the form of a checklist. At critical junctures in the procedures, the operator will need to sign and date the checklist to verify that the preceding steps have been carried out in accordance with the SOP. Alternatively, there can be two people involved in the assay. One person will carry out the steps of the assay, and the second will record and document that the steps were carried out appropriately. The second individual serves as the company's designated quality assurance/quality control monitor.

The SOP process takes on greater importance as products and procedures move into the realm of Good Laboratory Practices (GLPs) and Current Good Manufacturing Practices (cGMPs). The SOP is a fundamental building block in establishing a document record for FDA Investigational New Drug and Biologics License Applications. The SOPs are required throughout product development, from the preclinical and clinical processes to Chemistry, Manufacturing, and Controls (CMC) and safety evaluations.

chapter

13

•••••••••

HOW TO CHOOSE A POSTDOCTORAL POSITION

•••••••••••••••••

Having a career requires making decisions concerning the future. For many scientists, one of the critical branch points is determining where to complete a postdoctoral fellowship. There is often no single "right" or "wrong" choice but instead a wealth of excellent opportunities. So how do you select *one* postdoctoral position? This chapter outlines some of the elements to consider as you try to reach your answer.

DEFINE YOUR GOALS

For most of the life sciences, it is now routine for PhD graduates to complete at least one postdoctoral fellowship lasting from 2 to 4 years. Many young investigators will complete two postdoctoral positions before finding a full-time position in academia or industry. Whether you are a PhD student about to complete your thesis or a current postdoctoral fellow, the selection process is the same and can be summarized in one phrase: define your goals. One way to accomplish this is to discuss your career plans with your mentor, colleagues, friends, and family. These are the people who know you and who can serve as a sounding board for your ideas. It never hurts to get help when you are reaching an important decision. The systematic approach to this process that is described in this chapter should be a valuable tool when weighing your final decisions.

IDENTIFY YOUR SELECTION AND DECISION CRITERIA

Institutional

When deciding on a postdoctoral position, one area to consider is the kind of environment you want to work in. Institutional choices are abundant (see Table 13.1), and each type has unique features. Compared to the relatively protected time of your career in the postdoctoral period, institutional policies will most likely have a strong impact on you. Be sure to consider each institution's mission. A primary mission of all public universities is to serve the educational and economic needs of their state. Land grant universities have a close historical tie to the agricultural economy (consider land grant universities carefully if you are interested in using plant or large animal models). An objective at public university medical centers is to train the state's next generation of physicians and surgeons. In some states, this objective will impact the school's emphasis on basic science research activities as a priority across the campus. Private universities have unique missions, depending on their charter. Federal research laboratories serve the needs of the public at large and have congressionally mandated research

Table 13.1   Institutional Choices

Type of Institution	*Representative Example*
Land grant university	Oklahoma State University
Public university: basic science campus	University of Oklahoma—Norman
Public university: research center	Pennington Biomedical Research Center
Public university: medical center	University of Oklahoma Health Science Center
Public university: combined campus	University of Wisconsin—Madison (combined agriculture, basic science, and medical campus)
Private university: basic science campus	Princeton University
Private university: medical center	Baylor College of Medicine
Government research laboratory	National Institutes of Health
Nonprofit research foundation	Oklahoma Medical Research Foundation
Large pharmaceutical company	GlaxoSmithKline
Biotechnology company	Genentech

agendas. Nonprofit research foundations seek to achieve scientific excellence and cures for specific diseases, such as cancer. For-profit institutions must focus on drug design or product development, depending on their area of expertise.

Before choosing an institution type, also consider how the institution ties into the economy, because economic issues affect resource availability. Public universities have access to state funding, appropriated on an annual basis by the state legislature. When state tax revenues are reduced, funding levels can be severely impacted. Historically, land grant universities have access to strong support from the U.S. Department of Agriculture (USDA). Likewise, medical centers maintain close ties to funding from the National Institutes of Health (NIH), and basic science campuses receive grants from the National Science Foundation (NSF). Private universities and nonprofit research foundations usually have revenue-generating endowments and are the recipients of gifts from philanthropic organizations. In recent years, public universities have set up development offices to pursue private donations; nevertheless, such funds rarely account for a high percentage of a public institution's operating budget. In publicly traded, for-profit companies, product sales and stock values directly impact the operating costs allocated to research and development activities.

Cultural

Narrow your search process by determining what type of research you wish to pursue. Determine what you expect to gain from postdoctoral training at the technology or methodology level. What type of expertise will benefit your long-term career plans? What type of department do you wish to join? Different types of departments offer access to different technologies. For example, if you are interested in immunology, an immunology/rheumatology department at a medical center might provide access to primary human-based models; in contrast, a microbiology/immunology department at a basic science campus is more likely to provide access to simpler models, such as mice, drosophila, or nematodes.

Interpersonal

One of the most important issues to consider is with whom you will work. Your choice of a postdoctoral mentor and the way he or she runs the laboratory will have a major impact on how your own career will be molded. Consider your prospective mentor's educational background. What kind of credentials does he or she have? Did the mentor train as a PhD, an MD, a

DVM, a DDS, or some combination of degree programs? Where did the mentor receive training (in the United States or a foreign country, at a public or private institution, in a nonprofit or for-profit center)? These are the experiences that will shape the research activities and organization of the prospective mentor's laboratory. Each background offers unique advantages. If you trained as a PhD, working with a mentor from a clinical background will expose you to a different way of viewing a scientific question and how it should be pursued. Someone with a background in industry may have developed management/organizational skills that you can learn while on the job.

Everyone has different personalities, so consider if you and your mentor will be a compatible match. Ask yourself if the mentor is someone you can learn from and interact with on a routine basis. Look for a mentor who will give you the attention you need in a constructive and encouraging manner. The laboratory will reflect the personality of its leader, so look into the working environment for clues. Some people thrive where the postdoctoral fellows, students, and staff interact in a collegial manner. Others prefer to work in a more competitive arena, where two or more members of the laboratory are working independently on the same project. Choose the setting that best fits your own nature.

What is the productivity of the mentor's laboratory? This can be measured based on the mentor's publication record as determined by a

Table 13.2   Characteristics to Evaluate in a Potential Mentor

Graduate education	*DDS, DVM, MD, and/or PhD?*
Postdoctoral education	Where and when?
Private versus public experience	Government, industry, clinical, or other experience?
Personality	Is this someone you get along with? Do you respect him or her? Does he or she respect you?
Funding and publication track record	How often? Which journals? Quality? Authorship? Collaboration? Will you gain grant-writing experience?
Former trainee record	Do the mentor's former PhD students and postdoctoral fellows move on to positions you would want yourself? Did they have autonomy over their projects? Did they gain supervisory experience on the job?

PubMed search on the National Library of Medicine web site (http://www.ncbi.nlm.nih.gov/PubMed). Focus on the frequency of publications and the impact factor of the journals where these manuscripts appear. While there are legitimate criticisms concerning the formula calculating a journal's impact factor, university administrators routinely use this factor to "objectively" measure a scientist's productivity. Analyze the authorship profile of the mentor's average paper. Are the papers written by a single individual and the mentor, or are there multiple authors? Authorship will reflect how the mentor organizes collaborations among individuals within the laboratory and externally.

What resources does the mentor's laboratory command? This question cuts across institutional and cultural barriers. In concrete terms, it comes down to the actual infrastructure of the mentor's laboratory and the institution. Does the mentor's laboratory have state-of-the-art equipment sufficient to meet the research project's needs? Does the laboratory contain sufficient space to allocate a cubicle or desk to each postdoctoral fellow? How much space will you be able to use within the laboratory? Are there core facilities within the mentor's institution, such as gene microarray, proteomic, and transgenic mouse facilities? In intellectual terms, it comes down to the training infrastructure. Does the mentor's laboratory maintain a rotating schedule for data presentation and journal club among its staff? Are there one or more weekly seminar series on campus bringing in speakers relevant to the mentor's research activities? Are there funds available to attend national and/or international meetings in the mentor's field of research? Do you have access to a well-stocked brick and mortar library? Do you have access to a comprehensive electronic journal library? Do not take access to a wide array of journals for granted. Many smaller research institutions cannot afford the increasing cost of journal subscription and rely on interlibrary loan services for access to the literature. Be prepared to investigate this feature while exploring future postdoctoral positions.

In financial terms, investigate the mentor's external, federally funded grant record. This information is publicly available on the web pages of the NIH, NSF, USDA, and other agencies. The number and type of grants in the mentor's laboratory will give you some idea of the type of grant-writing experience you can expect to gain during your postdoctoral training. You need to find out if the postdoctoral training will include mentoring in "grantsmanship." In a laboratory within a private university medical center, you are likely to gain this experience; however, in a laboratory located at the NIH, a large pharmaceutical company, or a well-endowed private research foundation, you would be less likely to write an independent grant. In some laboratories, you will be expected to seek external funding to support your own salary. While this may appear to detract from the mentor's laboratory at first glance, it is also an opportunity. It is an indication that the mentor is committed to a culture of aggressively pursuing external funding at all levels and also that all members of the mentor's laboratory will receive hands-on grantsmanship experience.

Where do the mentor's former trainees wind up? This gives you some clues on how your own career might evolve. A mentor with close ties to industry may provide unique opportunities to trainees with an interest in moving into the for-profit sector. Other mentors may exclusively encourage trainees to pursue academic careers. If so, do these graduates spend the majority of their time in research or educational activities? If possible, contact current or former trainees from the mentor's laboratory. Just as the mentor will contact the references listed on your application, you can contact an equivalent set of references in reverse. It is important to address the degree of autonomy you will receive as a postdoctoral fellow. Autonomy is manifest at different levels and can be determined in part by asking the following questions: In terms of your project, does your mentor expect you to work on an existing protocol in the laboratory or to pursue an independent line of inquiry of your own choosing? Will the mentor expect you to work independently or cooperatively? Will you be able to draw on technical support from resources within the laboratory (i.e., will there be someone to wash glassware, prepare media and reagents, or to provide animal husbandry)? What will your responsibilities be within the laboratory? Will they include any teaching responsibilities in formal classes or supervisory duties for undergraduate and graduate students as well as research associates/technicians?

Personal

You are an individual with your own special needs. Intellectual factors may motivate your final decision when choosing a postdoctoral position. You

Table 13.3 Resources	
Tangible infrastructure	Laboratory equipment and space, office organization, and institutional core facilities
Intellectual infrastructure	Seminar series, opportunities to attend national and international meetings, journal subscriptions, and library
Funding infrastructure	Sources of external and internal funding, grant-writing opportunities, and expectations

Table 13.4	*Autonomy Survey*
Project selection	Is the project selected by the postdoctoral candidate alone or in consultation with the mentor? Or does the mentor assign it?
Project organization	Is the project organized by the postdoctoral candidate alone or in consultation with others, by the mentor alone, or by another process?
Technical support	What level is available? This can vary from no support to complete support.
Teaching responsibilities	Do you have formal teaching requirements in a classroom setting? Will you be training/supervising undergraduates, graduate students, research technicians, or other postdoctoral fellows?
Funding mechanism	Will you be required to submit a grant for your salary or research support? Will you contribute sections to grant applications from the laboratory?

may want to remain involved in the field of research that you pursued in your graduate thesis. Alternatively, you may want to branch out to a new area of research, to learn new technologies in different model systems. A wide range of personal issues will also affect your decision. A family member may have been diagnosed with a particular condition, motivating you at an emotional level to commit your energies to finding a cure. You may have geographic restrictions that will determine where you choose to take a postdoctoral position. Your significant other may have a position that requires you to locate in a particular part of the country. You may want to use your postdoctoral training period to experience living outside the United States. Or, you may have a family and need to find a location where you and your spouse are satisfied with the educational opportunities for your children. If you have a sick parent, you may wish to locate closer to his or her home. You may have financial obligations that require you to seek a position with a low cost of living and/or a high starting salary. Particular ideas on the size of the group you want to join could also influence your decision. You might seek out a large laboratory of more than 30 postdoctoral fellows or select a mentor who keeps a laboratory of less than 5 members. You may feel that you will deal better with a mentor at a particular stage of his or her career and of a particular gender. Although it is not politically correct to acknowledge either of these factors, they may influence your decision. All of these issues are personal and only you will know how they should be factored into the decision-making process.

Table 13.5 *Personal Decision Influences*	
Intellectual	***Old versus new field of research***
Geographic	To move or not to move (and how far)
Family	Single, married, and extended; how close or how far
Financial	Indebted or debt free; lifestyle concerns
Personal	Mentor's career stage, gender, and laboratory size

NEGOTIATING THE DEAL

Once you have evaluated a particular mentor and feel that a position may meet your needs, it is time to negotiate the details. It is recommended that you address several categories.

Intellectual

Determine what you can expect to gain intellectually in the position. For example, if your research evolves productively, will you be permitted to take a part of the research with you to your own independent laboratory? This has major implications on your ability to write a grant as a new faculty member following your postdoctoral training. In another example, if your mentor is a journal editor or reviewer, will you have the chance to learn how to critically review scientific manuscripts? This is a field of activity that you can best learn by doing, and you will benefit from such opportunities. Will you be able to learn techniques and/or pursue collaborations with neighboring laboratories within the mentor's institution or at external centers? These opportunities may vary, depending on the mentor and institution. For example, in a for-profit company, your opportunity to develop collaborations may be restricted by intellectual property concerns.

Determine what you are expected to give to the position. For example, what are the mentor's expectations for your productivity? How many manuscripts will you be expected to publish over a given time period? What type of journal will you be encouraged (and permitted) to publish in? In absolute terms, mentors can reasonably expect an average of one first-authored publication per year of postdoctoral fellowship. However, this value may be less if the mentor wants the postdoctoral publications to appear in *Nature*, *Cell*, or *Science*. Under these circumstances, it may take 2 or 3 years to develop a single publication. Some mentors refuse to publish in journals whose standards they do not respect or that fail to reach a particular scientific audience. Make sure that, prior to joining the laboratory, your expectations and those of your prospective mentor are in agreement on these issues. Will you be expected to write segments that will appear in grant applications, book chapters, or literature reviews? Will you be expected to present your work at national or international meetings? Will you be encouraged to give oral presentations of your work at these forums, or will oral presentations be at the perogative of the mentor? In each of these activities, you have the opportunity to save your mentor time and effort as well as to refine your own independent skills.

Temporal

Determine when your mentor expects you to arrive in the laboratory. Make sure this date gives you sufficient time to meet any of your prior commitments, such as the completion and defense of your PhD thesis. You are advised to complete your PhD requirements before entering your postdoctoral position. It is difficult to write and submit manuscripts with your thesis advisor while starting your postdoctoral research project. Also, it is rarely convenient to take vacation time within the first 3 months of your postdoctoral position in order to attend your graduation exercise; notify your prospective postdoctoral mentor in advance if this will be necessary.

Determine how long you can reasonably expect to stay in the laboratory. Neither you nor the mentor can cast this in stone. Nevertheless, it is helpful to have some idea of the degree of support that is currently allocated to your position. It is recommended that you secure a contract for at least 1 year and no longer than 3 years. This will provide you with both security and flexibility. It also gives both you and your mentor an idea on how soon you will need to devote time and energy to your next job hunting exercise.

Also determine how frequently you will meet with your mentor. This may take the form of group laboratory meetings or independent, one-on-one sessions between the two of you. These should be opportunities for you to review scientific as well as personal career issues during the course of your postdoctoral position. In addition, determine how frequently you will be expected or encouraged to present your data to the laboratory group and to other institutional seminar forums.

Financial

Last, but by no means least, is the issue of money. Determine what your base salary will be and whether it is negotiable. Some institutions have mandated a strict campus-wide pay scale for postdoctoral trainees based on education and years of experience. At other institutions, postdoctoral salary is determined at the discretion of the mentor. Determine if you can increase your salary by securing external grant support for the position. Some institutions provide an incentive to investigators who provide some or all of their salary through grant awards. Research how the negotiated salary compares to other postdoctoral positions at the same institution as well as at others like it in the same geographic region and nationally. Independent of the cost of living in a particular region, the salary level needs to be competitive on a national level. Ironically, you will sometimes find that institutions offering the highest postdoctoral salaries are located in geographic regions with the lowest costs of living. Such institutions may use this salary incentive as a recruiting tool. Consider the terms of the benefits package. Will you and your family receive health care benefits? Will you receive retirement and life insurance benefits? Will you and your family be eligible for reduced tuition payments for attendance in classes at your university employer? Finally, determine if you will receive reimbursement for any interviewing or moving expenses. Despite what you may have heard, it never hurts to ask about these topics, as long as you do it politely.

14

....

HOW TO CHOOSE A BIOTECHNOLOGY COMPANY

....

The process of moving into a biotechnology (or large pharmaceutical) company has analogous steps and stages to those you would use to find a postdoctoral position. You can apply the same strategy of analysis and ask many of the same questions, albeit in a somewhat different focus. There is one major difference to keep in mind. In choosing a postdoctoral position, your interpersonal relationship with your prospective mentor is probably the most important factor to consider. In choosing a biotech company, however, institutional and cultural considerations may prove of greater importance since personnel turnover is common in industry and it is impossible to predict how long any interpersonal relationship (either good or bad) will last.

DEFINING PERSONAL GOALS

Before anything else, take stock of your current situation. There are some very basic questions you need to ask yourself before embarking on a move from academia to biotech. Use your trusted friends, colleagues, and family members to help define your goals.

First, why are you leaving academia, and what do you want to accomplish in a biotech setting that you cannot do in academia? Evaluate your rationale dispassionately and objectively. In particular, focus on the scientific, intellectual, and financial advantages and disadvantages of each environment in relation to your current position. Scientifically, there are major differences between academia and biotech. It is important to appreciate the infrastructure that academia offers. A university medical center provides its investigators with access to vivariums as well as transgenic, microarray, proteomic, histology and other core facilities. Few biotech companies can match these multimillion-dollar resources. In biotech, you will need to develop strategic alliances or contracts with fee-for-service companies or with academic centers to obtain just a fraction of these resources. In academia, if you can obtain funding for a project, you are able to pursue it; rarely must you abandon a project before bringing it to some form of completion, either as a manuscript or thesis. Also in academia, the National Institutes of Health (NIH) and National Science Foundation (NSF) reach their funding decisions based on a scientific peer review panel. In biotech, however, venture capitalists, company executives, and/or stockholders who may or may not have a full appreciation of the scientific questions you hold dear often make funding decisions.

Secondly, when defining personal goals, are you prepared to deal with change? When I first joined a biotech company, an academic colleague summed up the difference in the two environments succinctly: "In academics, you measure time with a calendar; in biotech, you measure it with a stopwatch." Change occurs rapidly in the biotech arena. Executive and financial decisions can lead to priority changes in the research literally overnight. In biotech, you must be prepared to drop a project that has excellent scientific merit for nonscientific reasons that you may not fully understand. The scientific staff in biotech is not always privy to confidential information used to reach decisions behind closed doors in company boardrooms. It is difficult for many scientific investigators who have been principal investigators in control of their own academic laboratories not to be frustrated, angry, and bitter when faced with such situations in biotech. Intellectually and emotionally, if you are not prepared to deal with such a situation productively and to move on in step with the company's new focus, seriously consider whether you should move to biotech.

Finally, are you (and your family) prepared for an insecure future? When defining your personal goals, remember that jobs are far less stable in biotech than in academia. Even a soft money research professor position in academia is more secure than the position of chief scientific officer in a biotech company. In academia, the grant structure of a university allows you to predict when the money will run out; your salary is guaranteed for a 12-month period, and, unless you are fired for misconduct, you can be assured that the university will be able to keep its commitment to you through the expiration of your contract. At most universities, your job is protected by the strength of the faculty senate and, in some cases, by a union. In biotech, however, you are hired on a contract that can be cancelled at will. Few biotech companies are unionized. Private companies without sufficient venture capital funding may not be able to make payroll from month to month, leading to layoffs or liquidation of the entire company without prior notification to the general staff. In industry, you can estimate how long it will take to find an equivalent position based on your salary; it takes about 1 month for each $10,000. Thus, it may take a laid-off director-level scientist earning $120,000 approximately 1 year to find a similar position during a down market. The high salary structure in biotech relative to academia in part reflects the risk that the individual faces; you may need to have some of that money set aside in the event that you are unemployed for a period of time.

SELECTION CRITERIA

Once you have committed to making a move to biotech, it is time to do your research. There are several areas that you need to evaluate. To research effectively, complete a competitive analysis of companies with similar niche markets and/or that are located in the same geographic area.

Area of Research

It is important to find answers to several questions concerning the biotech company's area of research. What is the focus of the individual biotech company's research activity? Make sure that the company is pursuing a research strategy that is both scientifically and economically sound. If there are already major companies conducting the same or similar research, make sure that the biotech company you are considering has a competitive edge, either in the form of proprietary methods/data or intellectual property (patents). Does the research agenda fit with your individual goals? Make sure that the research is in an area that you can be excited about. You do not want to enter a company that is performing work that loses your interest immediately. How committed are the company's executives and board of directors to this area of research? Companies change their research focus for many reasons, and there are no guarantees for the future. Nevertheless, try to find out how long the company has pursued a particular project and how satisfied the management has been with its progress.

What other areas of research does the company have under development, and will they complement or compete with your own area of expertise or interest? A company that is committed to a single research program may be too narrowly focused to be successful. On the other hand, a company that is pursuing too many unrelated projects will never have the resources to do justice to them all. In such a circumstance, it is inevitable that some of those projects will have to be cut back or dropped. If you do join the company, one of your first jobs will be to promote the success of the project you join. You owe it to yourself to go into such a situation with your eyes open and to be aware of the possibility that the company management may need to address such concerns soon after you arrive on the scene. Will they present you with opportunities to learn, either at the technical or intellectual level? One way to view a new job is to look at it as preparation for your next job. Make sure you will acquire new skills and talents in your new position. This may come in the form of scientific expertise, such as an exposure to bioinformatics, or in a management capacity, such as the chance to be a project manager or team leader.

Company History

You will need to find out as much as possible about the company's record. Ask for a copy of the company's business plan or annual report if the information is not available on the company's web site. Look into the background of the company's founders and executive officers. Do they and their companies have a record of success? If so, what form does it take? In private companies, it is important to have a president and chief executive officer who is a successful fundraiser. This individual needs to have the ability and the connections to convince venture capital firms and investment banks to look favorably at the company's business plan. The extent of the company's intellectual property is critical; determine the number of issued and pending patent applications, review their publications, and find out whether they have projects at the preclinical, Phase I, Phase II, or Phase III level of development.

Does the company have an income-generating operation? Companies with profitable products or services have been more attractive to investors since the information technology (IT) bubble burst in 2001. If the company has undergone an initial public offering and is publicly traded, what has been the record of its stock value? The resources available for research are likely to rise and fall with the value of the company's stock. If the company is privately held, who are the major investors? Visiting the web sites of any investing venture funds can be enlightening. The venture firms will proudly display the names of other companies (past and current) that they have backed, with a description of their current level of success. You may discover that the venture capital funds that hold the majority of the company's stock have a long commitment to and interest in biotech and have a large reserve fund to use to support their companies (both good signs). Alternatively, you might find that the venture firm has invested in multiple companies in the IT sector that have done poorly and are draining the firm's limited resources. All of these facts will influence the company's stability as well as your future.

Degree of Autonomy

Once you begin interviewing, you need to determine how much control you will have over your own destiny. While it is likely that company management will establish the research goals, will you have input into the details of this agenda? Will you be able to publish, determine authorship on manuscripts initiated within your domain, have the opportunity to present your findings in public scientific forums, and collaborate and consult with academic colleagues? The answers to these questions will tell you a lot about the cultural climate within the biotech company. Some companies have a policy to retain all of their intellectual property in-house and refuse to share or distribute their findings except in the form of issued patents. Other companies view publications and meetings as a mechanism to advertise their progress and encourage investment. There are pros and cons to both approaches; however, it is likely that individuals coming directly from an academic environment will be more familiar with an open-door policy rather than a culture of secrecy.

Does the internal structure of the company's research program encourage collegiality and collaboration between groups, or does it promote competition for limited resources? Although the answer to this question may be hard to obtain, it will have a major impact on your work environment. Internal competition can be productive in a large company; in a small start-up, it is usually a scenario for disaster. Finally, is there an opportunity to pursue scientific questions outside the immediate interest of the company? It is unlikely that you will find this degree of autonomy in today's competitive environment outside of a few large pharmaceutical firms. If you do, it may reflect a biotech company with significant resources, tremendous confidence, and optimism for the success of its scientists. Alternatively, it could be a sign of poor management and a failure to understand the meaning of a for-profit research laboratory.

Resources

No matter how good ideas may be, you need to have the resources to turn them into data. What percentage of the company's annual budget goes into research activities and into your division in particular? Does the company have the equipment and instruments you will need to conduct your research? If not, can you use readily available subcontractors? Can you collaborate with university core laboratories through fee-for-service agreements, grants, or sponsored research agreements? Does the company have an existing relationship with the technology transfer office at the university? The cost of infrastructure is high. Many companies stretch their dollars by leasing equipment or buying time at university core laboratories. This presents a challenge because it requires you to shuttle your experiments across town or across the country. It can also cause delays if the university or company's legal offices have any concerns about intellectual property issues in such experiments.

Title

Shakespeare's quote about roses notwithstanding, the name of your position is very important. What will your title be, and how will it be perceived within the company's organization (org-chart) and externally? In some companies, the most senior and esteemed scientists are identified as "fellows"; in academia, someone with this title is likely to be recognized as a post-doc. Understanding your title will also tell you where you fall within the company's structure. This, in turn, determines where you stand in terms of access to information. If you report to a senior vice president, it is more likely that you will receive information about and have input concerning the company's policy decisions. On the other hand, if you report to a project leader or project director, you are farther removed from the company's policy center.

Salary and Benefits

At some point, it is time to get down to the nitty-gritty issues of paying your own bills. Will entry into the biotech arena meet your financial needs? Does the move represent an increase in your salary that is sufficient to offset the risks you face by leaving academia? Review what you will have in terms of health insurance coverage (medical and dental), disability insurance, and life insurance for yourself and your family. In addition, determine the form and extent of your retirement account and the company's contribution to it; you need to assess the pros and cons of stock options in light of the current market situation.

When considering salary and benefits, there are other features to evaluate. If you are going to lose a retirement bonus, such as a 5-year vesting plan, by leaving your current position, will the biotech company purchase it for you as a moving incentive? What form will your salary take: a base salary, annual year-end bonuses based on the ability of your division to achieve corporate milestones, and/or bonuses determined by your supervisor based on your personal performance? Will you receive stock options upon joining the company? If so, will your stock options be determined by your rank or by a formula linked to your starting salary?

CULTURAL LEVEL

Each company has its own distinct culture. In some companies, the management team has specific ideas about the company culture and has taken active steps to foster and encourage certain corporate behaviors at the institutional level. In other companies, the culture simply reflects the personalities of the founders and initial leaders within the various departments. In evaluating a biotech company, you need to understand what the company's culture is like, how it evolved, and whether you can comfortably fit into it.

Look first into the history of the company and its founders. For companies based on intellectual property from academic laboratories and developed within incubators attached to academic centers, the culture is likely to resemble that of a university laboratory. This is particularly true if the founders are university professors who continue to maintain their academic ties. These founders will emphasize research and discovery rather than development and manufacturing since this is what they are most familiar with. Personnel will not be expected to follow a dress code, report to work at a specified time, and follow a strict organizational hierarchy. For companies founded by former scientists and directors in large pharmaceutical companies, the culture will be geared more to a big-business model. Emphasis, resources, and rewards will be distributed equally between research and development, manufacturing, regulatory, and sales departments. Attention to personal appearance, regular work hours, and "chain of command" management structures will be more common features of the workplace. The biotech culture may appear more "buttoned up" compared to the academic environment you may be familiar with.

The nature of the company's financial backing will also influence its culture. In start-up companies funded by *family and friends*, emotional factors will impact the company's culture. Under such circumstances, the founders will be concerned about their personal commitments to their investors not as businessmen but as relatives. No matter how the company performs, this investor–founder relationship will continue to have a direct effect on the culture you join.

In start-up companies funded by *venture capitalists*, the history of the venture firm and its record of success (or failure) are worth considering. Some venture firms take a hands-off approach to their biotech companies; others micromanage, taking a direct interest in the day-to-day operation and finances. In part, the venture firm's involvement will reflect its confidence in the company's management team and the strength of personality of the company's leadership.

In *publicly traded* companies, the company's culture will be significantly different. The Securities and Exchange Commission (SEC) mandates certain accounting and monitoring practices for public companies that will trickle down to all levels of the company's culture. These will involve more sophisticated levels of documentation, greater attention to public statements, and greater levels of security consciousness on the part of the staff.

You should also take other financial matters into consideration. If a company has just emerged from a significant loss in income, you may encounter a depressed and demoralized staff, particularly if layoffs have occurred. Alternatively, if a company has just landed a major contract, released a new product, or successfully completed a major Phase III trial, you may encounter a staff brimming with optimism and confidence.

It is worthwhile to look at the company's lifespan and maturation. Does the company have products on the market, in the pipeline, or in its dreams? In a mature company with marketable products, you will encounter a culture in which management will value the sales force as highly as any other entity within the company. Their activities will directly drive profits and revenues. Because research efforts need time to generate profits directly, your scientific activities may not be held in high esteem in such a culture. In contrast, in a start-up company, research activity will play a greater role and will receive a greater percentage of the company's resources. For better or worse, management will pay greater attention to the company's research activities and productivity.

INTERPERSONAL LEVEL

In biotech, your interpersonal relationships hold less importance than in academia. Turnover in business is rapid, and the people you meet during your interviews may be gone by the time you arrive as an employee. Nevertheless, gauge the chemistry you feel between the company personnel and yourself. How do you relate to your immediate supervisor and the senior management of the company? What kind of rapport do you sense between yourself and your peers and direct reports? Even though these impressions are subjective, they deserve your attention and consideration.

If your gut feeling says there is something wrong at this level, you may want to revisit your objective criteria in evaluating the company. These may be signs that this is not the appropriate setting in which to risk your future.

NEGOTIATIONS

Negotiations will take place throughout the interview process. Be aware of this and be prepared to request specific information and requirements before you make a commitment to join a biotech company. After you have signed on as an employee, you will have lost most of your negotiating strength. A company's representatives have a primary obligation to serve the interests of the corporation—not those of potential employees. While the company's management most likely desires to create an environment that supports the welfare of its employees, you need to advocate your own interests and goals. Most items on the agenda (salary, benefits, title, etc.) are negotiable within a range of values. Chances are that you have been offered an amount that is less than or equal to the midpoint of that range. You can remain professional and still request that any element of your package be increased or altered. Do your homework and make sure you receive an offer that is competitive with similar companies in the field and for equivalent positions in that geographic area. Routinely, you should not take a new position without achieving some financial reward, preferably represented by a cost-of-living salary increase of more than 10% of your current salary.

EXIT STRATEGY

Whenever a venture firm considers an investment in a start-up company, it does so with an exit strategy in mind. The investors have a clear idea of how and when they expect to benefit from the investment. You should do the same. Determine what you want to obtain by joining the biotech company. Identify particular skills, competencies, and milestones you expect to realize. Make sure you have a clear idea of how the job you accept will train you for your next position in industry or academia.

Biotech companies have a lifespan consisting of different stages. If you are particularly interested in research, you might enjoy working in an early stage biotech company; however, as the company matures and brings its science into the development, clinical, and marketing stages, you may find the environment less engaging. Of course, your interests may change as you are exposed to different opportunities and challenges. You may discover that you find elements of the U.S. Food and Drug Administration (FDA) regulatory process challenging and decide to pursue issues relating to Good Laboratory Practice (GLP) and current Good Laboratory Practice (cGMP) as you grow with the company. Regardless, keep a flexible outlook and be aware that life in biotech is uncertain. Maintain contacts with colleagues and friends concerning other opportunities. When companies close, the process can be rapid and unexpected. You want to keep an up-to-date resume handy to be able to rapidly and efficiently cope with unforeseen circumstances.

15

· · · · · · · · · ·

HOW TO SET UP
A LABORATORY

· · · · · · · · · · · · · · · · ·

Your laboratory's structure will impact your productivity and success as long as you occupy it. There have been many excellent books written on how to set up a laboratory. This chapter draws on them to briefly describe some of the elements you should consider as you build your own.

ORGANIZING

There is one fundamental tenet to the process of building a laboratory: organization. How you organize your resources in preparation for your new laboratory will be directly reflected in the final outcome. You and the people who work with you will either reap the benefits of your planning or pay the consequences of your ensuing chaos. Whatever you decide to do will set a precedent for the future growth and development. If you expect to expand your laboratory in the future, provide a framework that has the necessary flexibility to accommodate this growth. No matter what resources you command, they will always be limited (and never enough!). Use them wisely.

INVENTORIES

In the computer age, it is easy to organize and update your inventories using spreadsheets. Take full advantage of this capability from the start.

By establishing appropriate inventory methods and processes before you open your laboratory, you can generate a complete record of your laboratory's assets that grows with you. A list of inventories to consider is presented in Table 15.1. These inventories will serve multiple purposes, including (1) a record for you and your personnel, allowing easy access to

Table 15.1 Inventories	
Category	*Content*
Chemical	Chemical name, CAS number, vendor/supplier, catalog number, electronic link to Material Safety and Data Sheet (MSDS), storage condition (room temperature, $4°$ or $-20°$ C), date obtained, shelf life
Plasmids	Identification number, vector name, insert (cDNA identification, species of origin), vector properties (antibiotic resistance, map), source of plasmid (investigator name, institution, contact information), reference (journal citation), date of entry, name of lab member who prepared the plasmid
$-80°$ C freezer contents	Location (shelf number, box number), content, date of entry, name of lab member entering data
Liquid nitrogen storage contents	Location (shelf number, box number), cell type, cell concentration, volume per vial, date of entry, name of lab member entering data
Radioactive materials	Radioisotope, chemical composition, vendor, catalogue number, reference date for half-life determination, utilization history, disposal history (solid, liquid, drain), remaining isotope on hand, date of entry, name of lab member entering data
Tissue specimens	Tissue, specie, experiment or patient subject reference, date of harvest, date of entry, record of utilization, storage type (paraffin embedded, in ethanol, frozen at $-20°$, $-80°$, or liquid nitrogen)
Notebooks	Identification number, date notebook issued, individual to whom notebook issued, date notebook completed, storage location of notebook, contents
Reports and documents	Document/file name, authors, date of completion, date, identity of record keeper

past data and resources; (2) a record for future personnel who may replace you, including future owners of the company; (3) a mechanism for evaluating and documenting components of the laboratory for safety, regulatory compliance, and value; and (4) added value to the assets of the company in the event of a sale or liquidation.

EQUIPMENT AND MANUALS

It is equally important to maintain accurate and up-to-date records on equipment. No matter which model or brand you purchase, every equipment item will malfunction at some point in its history. And, if Murphy's Law has anything to do with it, it will be at the worst possible time. Whenever a malfunction occurs, easy access to the equipment records and service requirements will help improve what is invariably a troublesome situation. Your records should be established when the equipment is purchased and installed. Consider inclusion of the following information in your records:

- Equipment item name
- Manufacturer (with location and contact information)
- Model number
- Serial number
- Warranty information
- Date of purchase
- Certification record and history
- Service history (list any repairs, malfunctions, replaced parts)
- Record of routine maintenance (list performance date and identification of service personnel or staff responsible)

All equipment comes with a service manual. Determine how frequently and how thoroughly you need to perform preventive maintenance. Think of it like your automobile: would you run a car for 10,000 miles without checking (or changing) your oil? If you would, you may want to consider an alternative operating procedure for your laboratory or find a way to pass this responsibility to someone else who is more detail oriented and machine friendly than yourself. Provide your laboratory with a centralized repository for all equipment manuals. Locate this within the domain of the person (or persons) who will be overseeing any future repairs or maintenance.

METHODS, PROTOCOLS, AND STANDARD OPERATING PROCEDURES

You and your laboratory will have proprietary methods and protocols unique to your area of research. Together, they are a valuable resource. Organize these items electronically, categorizing them into folders associated with selected areas such as "Molecular Biology," "Cell Biology," "Histology," and so forth. Some would argue that such records should be identified solely by an abbreviated letter code (such as CB for Cell Biology) and a three-digit number. This discourages someone without authorization from easily rifling through the files. A more user-friendly title, however, is one that can be easily searched and identified by name (such as "CB001 – Isolation of Adult Stem Cells from Murine Bone Marrow). While this allows an external auditor to access and cross-reference records (not always a desirable feature), it also simplifies searches by laboratory personnel. Before implementation of an inventory system, your company will need to weigh the pros and cons of a user-friendly versus a security-conscious system.

REFERENCES

Barker, K. *At the Helm: A Laboratory Navigator*. Cold Springs Harbor, NY: Cold Springs Harbor Laboratory Press, 2002.

Barker, K. *At the Bench: A Laboratory Navigator*. Cold Springs Harbor, NY: Cold Springs Harbor Laboratory Press, 2002.

Blumberg, D. D., and Zoon, R. A. Requirements for a molecular biology laboratory. *Methods in Enzymology* **152**, 3–32, 1987.

16

· · · · · · · · · ·

HOW TO ADMINISTER
A LABORATORY

· · · · · · · · · · · · · · · · ·

Once you have laid the foundation of your laboratory, the next challenge is to run it. This will draw on all of your scientific knowledge and training. In addition, it will call for you to develop and use personnel management skills, which are usually taught in business schools. Chances are, you never took those classes. This chapter introduces some of these concepts in the context of a laboratory environment.

PERSONNEL

Recruitment of Personnel

Your laboratory will only be as good as the people working with you. Part of this will be determined by who you recruit. The rest will reflect how you train your personnel after they are working with you. To recruit, you will need to exploit all of the available pipelines and professional networks. Consider applicants from local, national, and international sources. The local talent pool is less expensive to bring on board and may have local connections of value to the laboratory, such as direct knowledge of your institution's operating systems. National and international recruits may bring specialized training and talents that complement your existing operation.

International candidates will require additional paperwork for immigration and naturalization requirements. In the post-9/11 world, this burden has increased significantly. As a result, the time frame for the arrival of an international candidate can take 6 months to a year or more. Even after his or her arrival, there may be lost periods of productivity due to lapses in paperwork and a loss of work-visa status.

To identify the right people, you will need sophisticated interviewing skills. Before beginning, talk to your human resources (HR) officer or personnel director for suggestions and guidance. Remember, there are certain questions you cannot ask in any interview (Table 16.1). Try not to make mistakes in this process, no matter how innocent, that you may have to pay for later. Much of the "forbidden information," such as dates of birth, citizenship, and country of origin, is routinely included in the resumes and curriculum vitae of most academic candidates. Nevertheless, that does not mean you are legally allowed to request that information directly.

Determine the personnel you need in your laboratory. Consider your budget and who is available. Consider also the ratio you want to maintain between undergraduate students, graduate students, postdoctoral fellows, research assistants/technicians, instructors, research assistant faculty members, or their equivalents. Define (on paper) a detailed job description for each position. Provide in broad terms a list of the job's responsibilities, performance expectations, reporting structure, educational requirements, and prior experience level. These documents can be further customized if a particular skill set is specifically required; otherwise, they can be used without editing whenever a position at a particular level opens up.

Always ask for and check references from individual candidates. Word of mouth is often the best way to find and check qualified applicants. The best references, from your viewpoint, will come from individuals you already know. Hopefully, the references will give you an accurate and honest appraisal of the candidate. Records of references will be accessible to the candidate if they take legal steps to obtain them. This fact is likely to inhibit the candor of some reference letters. Therefore, pay as much attention to what is not said in a letter of recommendation as to what is said. While a failure to comment on a candidate's interpersonal skills may just be a sign of a poorly written reference letter, it can also be a very important clue. The reference may be implying that this individual did not get along with his or her peers and was a disruptive member of the team. Sometimes a phone conversation to a reference with some carefully phrased questions can be helpful. In such a circumstance, it would be useful to ask parallel questions, such as "How would you assess this candidate's ability to work (a) independently, and (b) with others as a contributing member of the team?" The responses

Table 16.1   *What You Can and Cannot Ask in an Interview*

Subject Area	Can Ask	Cannot Ask
Nationality	Are you legally allowed to work in the U.S.? What languages are you fluent in?	Are you a U.S. citizen? Where were you born? What is your native language?
Personal	Are you able to perform the following physical tasks on the job?	How tall are you? How much do you weigh?
Age	Are you over the age of 18?	How old are you? What is your birthdate? When did you graduate from college?
Family	Would you relocate? Are you willing to travel on the job? Can you work overtime/weekends?	What is your marital status? Who lives with you? Do you plan to have children? How many children do you have?
Disabilities	Can you perform the essential activities of the job? (You can require the candidate to undergo a medical exam for the job.)	Do you have any disabilities? Have you had any recent illnesses? How is your family's health? When did you lose a physical ability?
Arrest record	Have you ever been convicted of a particular crime?	Have you ever been arrested?
Military record	In what branch of the military did you serve? What type of training/ education did you receive in the military?	If you were in the military, were you honorably discharged?
Affiliations	Do you belong to any organizations relevant to performance of this job?	What organizations/ social clubs do you belong to?

are likely to address any doubts you may have about the individual's suitability for your own laboratory.

Not all job candidates can or will be open in their selection of references. Some employers are threatened when personnel look at alternative positions. In some instances, employers reduce the responsibility level of or fire employees who have pursued other job opportunities. Therefore, you should not insist on references from a current employer. Of course, do not ever expect a candidate to knowingly give you a "bad" reference. Applicants have the ability to preselect the list of references and should do so to their own maximum advantage. Consequently, when and if you do receive a less-than-positive reference on a candidate, you should take the message very seriously. It is likely that a former employer or colleague is doing you a favor.

Hiring

Determine the protocol for hiring with your human resources officer. For example, if your advertisement for a position included a requirement for a master's degree under educational experience, you may discover that you cannot hire the best candidate who applies only because he or she has a bachelor's degree and 15 years of experience instead of a master's degree. Work out this level of detail in advance. Furthermore, delegate issues regarding benefits, vacation time, and even salary to the human resources personnel whenever possible. By doing this, you keep some potentially difficult issues at an institutional level and avoid having them become interpersonal-level areas of conflict. Ultimately, it is in your best interests to be familiar with your company's or institution's employee manual and personnel policies.

Performance Review Process

Within the first month after hiring a new employee, you should discuss the performance review process with him or her. This is designed to be a proactive development plan to meet your needs as well as the employee's needs. It has the capacity and flexibility to maintain effective and consistent communication and to reduce the development of problems in the future. Within this framework, focus on the positive issues first. It is advisable to always present your praises before your criticisms. Identify the strengths the employee brings to the new job. Be sure to keep a balance in your evaluation process by not giving false praise in the expectation that it will improve performance.

The next step is to discuss areas in which you and the employee would like to seek growth in the employee's new role. Try to develop a consensus in identifying these areas. You are more likely to encourage an honest effort and development from your employees if they "buy in" to the area(s) in which they need to improve their performance.

Table 16.2 contains a list of competencies and skills to use as an aid to the performance review process. This list includes specific areas to evaluate that are related to setting objectives, leadership, resource management, interpersonal skills, communication, adaptability, and team building. Focus on one or two items for the immediate future (3–4 months). Then implement and maintain a set schedule of meetings to review performance development. Be sure to document goals and milestones for improvement and development. This record, which you and the employee should prepare together, will monitor the individual's success (or lack thereof) in meeting the identified and agreed-upon competencies and skills. By keeping a clear line of communication throughout the process, you will avoid any misunderstanding in the event that the employee's performance falls short of expectations. If an employee proves to be unsatisfactory, performance review records will play a major role in determining whether you are able to remove the employee from the position.

Even if you are not completing a formal performance review, do not fail to acknowledge and appreciate satisfactory or better levels of performance. These positive remarks should be shared in the context of specific job outcomes. For example, instead of waiting 2 months until a scheduled performance review to tell an employee that the job he or she did was outstanding, give praise right away. Furthermore, let your employee know that you will remember his or her excellent work when the formal performance review comes around later.

Table 16.2   Competencies and Skills

Competency or Skill	Evaluation Question
Setting direction	Is this person a problem solver?
Leadership	Can you rely on this person to take charge?
Selection of people	Does this person recruit competent colleagues to your team?
Development of people	Can this person be an effective mentor?
Management of resources	How well does this person work within your budget?
Communication skills	Can this person be a public spokesperson for a project?
Teamwork	Can this person build an effective project team?
Adaptability	Is this person flexible in a changing environment?
Situation knowledge	Does this person understand your priorities?

As part of the initial performance development review, build a contract with your supervisee. Be sure to build specific contracts for undergraduate and graduate students, postdoctoral fellows, research technicians, and faculty members. At the same time, have the employees identify what they expect from the job and from you as a supervisor. In return, you need to be prepared to outline both what they expect from you and what you expect from them. Make it clear what you intend to do for your employees, but do not make promises you cannot keep or guarantee. However, try to strive to deliver above and beyond anything you do actually promise.

Establishing a Laboratory Culture

Individual laboratories have distinct cultures. Some operate as an umbrella for a group of individuals who are all striving for excellence on their own particular projects, usually with varying degrees of success. Others are team-oriented with clear-cut areas of specialization for individuals and coordinated projects shared by many. As the laboratory's leader, your style will influence the direction of the culture. Some laboratory leaders recruit individuals who are already trained in a particular discipline and technique. These new hires are then assigned projects that are ripe for the application of their unique expertise.

Other laboratory leaders create an atmosphere of cross-fertilization and technique development. Any member of the laboratory can approach any other member for instruction and assistance in a particular method. Such collaborations are encouraged and fostered from the highest level within the laboratory and are rewarded with coauthorship on manuscripts where appropriate. Likewise, some leaders encourage their staff to be fearless in attempting new techniques and adapting assays from the literature or other laboratories to their projects. These approaches can lead to a self-sustaining and empowering scientific environment. Instead of needing to recruit individuals with specialized skills and talents, you can develop expertise in-house as it is required. Leaders of such a laboratory are less likely to lie awake at night worrying about where they will find the next best postdoctoral candidate. There will be a greater sense of self-confidence that personnel who have demonstrated mastery of one method can be trained or, even better, self-taught to master another.

Shared Responsibilities

It is tempting to hire individuals solely as support staff. If an operation reaches a sufficiently large size, it makes economic sense to hire someone to wash dishes, prepare media/buffers, and to maintain the tissue culture room for everyone else. However, one of the risks of having a laboratory "maid" is that the remaining personnel take this service for granted and become sloppy and wasteful in their experimental habits. You will find that people pay closer attention to what they use and how they clean up if they are held responsible for the appearance and stocking of the laboratory. Equipment maintenance improves when everyone shares the job of checking and cleaning equipment. You are less likely to break an instrument if you are fully trained and aware of how it can malfunction in its operation. To achieve this goal, you should establish a responsibility list that involves all members of the laboratory (students, postdoctoral fellows, technicians, and even faculty members). Table 16.3 provides an example of a responsibility list. New members of the laboratory should be immediately included in the process. To prevent anyone from acquiring an undesirable job, rotate the responsibilities on a regular basis (every 3 or 6 months); this will also ensure that everyone has an opportunity to work with multiple aspects of the laboratory's infrastructure over time.

To monitor these activities, it is helpful to have a maintenance record form on a clipboard or in a notebook located in the immediate vicinity of the equipment. Likewise, an electronic inventory of these activities is useful.

Micromanaging

One of the most difficult adjustments to leadership is allowing yourself to delegate tasks to others. There are many tasks that you will feel you can do more

Table 16.3   Laboratory Responsibility List for Cell/Molecular Biology Laboratory

Chore	Frequency
Clean/check water baths	Weekly
Clean/check CO_2 incubators	Weekly
Clean biological safety cabinets	Weekly
Remove/autoclave biohazard waste	Daily
Monitor radiation safety records and area	Monthly
Maintain supply inventory	As needed
Maintain liquid nitrogen cell storage facility	Weekly
Maintain balances and pH meter	As needed
Maintain −80° C freezers	Weekly
Maintain centrifuges	Quarterly
Wash/autoclave glassware	Daily

quickly than a new graduate student or technician. The challenge is to have the patience to stand back and let others take over. Remember, even after new employees have received suitable and appropriate instruction, it is common for them to make unintentional mistakes. If you have hired well, your employees' conscience and desire to achieve will do more to spur them on to a better performance than anything you can add. Therefore, do everything you can to control your temper and give them the opportunity to try again with your full encouragement. Even if the employees never perform the task as fast as you can, their efforts will save you time in the long run. Remember, it is impossible to do everything yourself. The goal is to fill your laboratory with people who can do the tasks as well as or better than you could yourself. Over time, you will find that any tendency you have to micromanage your staff will be replaced by an admiration for their performance and competence. It may even give you pause to wonder about your own contribution to the effort and whether the success of the laboratory is due to or in spite of your management practices. These may be questions that are better left unanswered except in the privacy of a beer, a bar, and the ear of a good friend.

FINANCES

When administering a laboratory, finances are just as important as your personnel. Science is an expensive undertaking no matter how and where it is studied. Ultimately, someone pays for everything that is done in your institution. Make sure you know what you will need to pay for each year, where the money will come from, and whether you can afford it.

Budget Preparation

You can view your budget from a temporal perspective. In grant applications, you will plan budgets for a particular project and over a period of several years. At the institutional level, you will likely have to work within an annual operating budget for your entire laboratory or department. To monitor your activity, you will probably watch the money flow on a month-by-month basis. To facilitate this, you should proactively determine what level of average monthly expenditure you can afford; attach a set dollar amount to this level. If you observe that costs in any given month are going to exceed this value, look into your laboratory's economy and determine the cause of this. Also ask whether further changes in purchases or usage should be mandated.

One simple way to make sure your money is used effectively is to make everyone aware of the costs of their own operation. You should not be surprised to learn that students and postdoctoral fellows do not know how much it really costs to run just one of their experiments. Let each of your personnel develop a budget (including their salary and fringe benefits) for their experiments on an annual basis. They will probably exercise a more conservative approach to their spending habits if they know what it costs to keep them gainfully employed and productive.

Costs get out of control if multiple personnel in the laboratory are ordering independently. This leads to duplicate purchases, the use of expensive vendors, excessive back inventory, and redundant shipping costs. Centralize ordering responsibilities to a single individual such as a laboratory manager or purchasing officer. Define a threshold or cutoff limit for all orders that will require your direct approval. Below these limits, give the laboratory manager autonomy and responsibility. Of course, this can only be done if you provide and maintain effective oversight on a timely basis. You should meet weekly or monthly with your purchasing agent to review orders and expenditures. The frequency of these meetings will depend on the size and scope of your laboratory's average expenditures.

Budgets can be problematic when they are too small or too large. If times are lean, you may be tempted to do too many things without sufficient resources (there are always so many exciting unsolved scientific questions to address). While it is important to meet milestones, do not retain goals that are unrealistic due to unforeseen expenses. Take the tough steps to cut back and focus your limited resources on achievable and critical goals. Make sure you can define product-oriented goals within your budget. In academia, it will not advance your research efforts to reach an intermediate stage on two separate projects if you fail to publish a manuscript on either study. In biotechnology, you will not advance your company's product by pursuing two preclinical trials simultaneously if by doing so you cannot move either one to the clinical stage of development.

If money is abundant, do not allow yourself or your team to become fiscally undisciplined. No one will reward you for waste. It will be that much more difficult to instill a thrifty economy in your laboratory when adjustments from the accounting office force you to "normalize" your budget and expenditures in the future. Poor spending habits are problems that are always difficult to correct.

You do not need to be an accountant to successfully run a laboratory under a budget. Instead, you need to be familiar with several terms that are introduced below.

Direct costs

Direct costs refer to the cost of services and goods required for a project. Remember, the cost of a chemical is not simply the list cost in the catalog, but it also includes the fee for shipping and handling (such as the inclusion of dry ice in the container) and markups due to any intermediary (such as an institution's on-site store and ordering agent).

Indirect costs

Institutions receiving federal grants or contracts routinely negotiate an *indirect cost* rate with the government. These fees are designed to cover institutional infrastructure expenses, such as electricity, plumbing, and building maintenance, that are not included as direct costs on a grant. Indirect cost rates can be anywhere from 40 to 100% or more of the direct costs of the grant. Levels vary with the size and scope of the institution's operation as well as its location. Indirect cost rates in major urban centers (New York, Boston, San Francisco) are generally greater than those in less congested areas (Iowa City, Oklahoma City, Tucson). Private research foundation grants may cap indirect costs at a rate of 10% or less; some foundations allow none.

Many institutions and departments share indirect costs with the laboratories of individual investigators. A percentage of the indirect costs recovered on a principal investigator's grants may be returned to his or her department or laboratory directly by the dean of the college or other institutional authority. Sometimes, this comes in the form of a salary bonus to act as an incentive to encourage future successful grant applications. Alternatively, the sum may be in the form of additional funds for research support. This may be directly paid to the investigator's laboratory or applied through indirect mechanisms. For example, indirect costs may be used to offset the cost of operating a core facility within the institution; reduced usage fees thereby benefit all of the institution's researchers and the budgets of their individual laboratories.

Salaries and fringe benefits

Many institutions have strict guidelines and salary ranges for specific job descriptions and categories. As an assistant professor in the life sciences, there is probably a salary cap that you can only exceed by promotion to an associate professor level. Be familiar with the guidelines within your institution. Most state institutions are required to make salaries for individual faculty members part of the public record. Do not be surprised if there is an occasion on which you read about your own salary (and those of your colleagues) on the front page of your local newspaper. You should know how your institution's average salary levels compare to other institutions at the regional and national levels. If you want to recruit the best people to your laboratory, you need to meet or beat the salary offered by competitors. This information is available through annual surveys and is often published in *Science, The Scientist,* and other journals.

Salaries are more than just the actual wages that employees directly receive. They also include fringes, which are hidden costs to the institution and, ultimately, to your laboratory. Fringe benefits include health insurance, retirement plan contributions, life and disability insurance policies, social security contributions, and educational benefits to the employee, spouse, and children. These are calculated either as a flat percentage of the employee's base salary or as a sliding percentage of the salary. Depending on income, the sliding scale percentage can be as high as 40% for a low income wage earner to about 20% for an executive or full professor in a clinical department.

Salary levels can also be evaluated based on the cost of living in your city/locale. A dollar in Des Moines is worth more for real estate property than a dollar in Manhattan. Nevertheless, do not be deceived. You may still need to pay the same or more to recruit a highly qualified individual to a less expensive region of the country. Many job candidates on the East and West Coasts are reluctant to leave the perceived benefits of their densely populated urban centers for the perceived cultural disadvantages of a Midwestern or Southern destination. You may only be able to attract these employees by offering them a salary well above the immediate prospects offered in their current locale.

Service costs

Many *service costs* fall between the budgeting categories listed so far. These include equipment maintenance costs, contracts, repair fees, and replacement costs. Some of these fees can be included in grants. Costs for secretarial support, phones, faxes, Internet services, courier shipments, postage, and other expenditures are more difficult to recover. Even though there may not be a specific grant to pay for these services, you will always need them. Somehow, your budget will reflect these costs.

PUBLICATION EXPECTATIONS

As you develop your laboratory, set down your criteria for publication expectations as a measure of productivity. Introduce this concept to new employees to establish an intra-laboratory culture of excellence. Identify the average frequency of publication authorship you expect from individuals on your team at their particular job level (see Table 16.4). Likewise, prepare a list of suggested journals in which you would prefer to see your manuscripts published. Rate these based on your assessment of them as initial submission targets or as secondary submission targets following any rejections. Journal selection will reflect the area of expertise and research focus of your laboratory. You should strive to publish in the leading top five journals in your field as a primary goal. Those journals with the widest audience of your peers and those outside your immediate field are the optimal (and usually the most selective) targets. You can and should use the ISI Web of Knowledge impact factor rating as a guide to selection and evaluation of journals for publications (http://www.isiwebofknowledge.com/index.html). While there is controversy concerning the use of this information, it remains a valuable and commonly used rating tool by scientists and administrators in both academia and biotech.

LEAVING THE LABORATORY

It is important to leave your laboratory to run itself from time to time. This has two major benefits: (1) it gives you a break from the day-to-day routine, and (2) it gives your laboratory a chance to appreciate your presence and to develop its self confidence. There is no question that your presence is important to the running of your laboratory; however, you should not be indispensable to its operation. Your staff should be capable of maintaining an acceptable level of productivity in your absence. You can only prove this to everyone concerned by putting a little distance between yourself and the laboratory. Once you take a few trips away from the laboratory, everyone will develop a routine to anticipate your absence as well as mechanisms to deal with any issues that might need attention while you are gone.

Meetings

It is critical that you travel to national and international meetings on a regular basis. These opportunities to network with colleagues allow you to

Table 16.4 Publication Expectations		
Position	*Average Number of Annual First-Author Publications*	*Average Number of Annual Contributing-Author Publications*
Undergraduate	0	0.5
Graduate (1–2 yr)	0	0.5–1
Graduate (3–5 yr)	1	0.5–1
Postdoctoral fellow	1	1–2
Assistant technician	0	1
Senior technician	0	≥ 2
Instructor	1	1

inform others of your work, to meet with members of study sections from granting agencies, and to learn about unpublished research findings from other laboratories in your field. If your budget allows, attend a minimum of two to four meetings annually. Submit an abstract to each meeting, and request an oral presentation whenever possible. Find an international society in your field of research, and attend its annual meeting regularly. Use the society's journal as a forum for your publications on a regular basis. By doing so, you will discover that your own work becomes better known among the society's members and they will become your friends and collaborators throughout your career.

Sabbaticals

Academia and biotech often allow faculty-level staff to take sabbaticals of 1–12 months in length after a period of uninterrupted service; however, only a minority of eligible faculty take advantage of the perk. Despite all the reasons not to disrupt the routine of your laboratory and your life, take the sabbatical. It is amazing how much you can learn from a visit away from home. The change of venue is invigorating and enlightening. You can use sabbaticals to learn new technologies, develop new collaborations, and recruit young colleagues back to your own laboratory. A sabbatical can be a time for personal growth for you and your family. By scheduling a sabbatical in a foreign country, you can experience another culture both inside and outside the laboratory.

It is interesting to visit another university department or corporate system as a privileged outsider. You can observe how that organization functions without having any major responsibility for its operation. You can see how the host institution differs from your parent organization and discover new models that can be adapted to your own laboratory or institution upon your return. Of course, it will also be a time to weigh the merits and demerits of your current position and situation. Upon completion, your sabbatical may give you a greater appreciation of the assets and benefits you receive from your university or company. Alternatively, the sabbatical may give you a wake-up call and motivate you to explore new career opportunities.

Seminars

Most institutions have some form of a seminar series. Take advantage of these resources to invite current or potential collaborators and leaders in your field to visit your institution. Whenever a colleague visits, be a good host. Make sure to provide him or her with a schedule that meets everyone's needs and is not exhausting. Try to schedule visits with as many of your institution's faculty and staff members as possible. One-on-one meetings should be 30–45 minutes in length. In general, too little time in these meetings is better than too much. It is preferable that colleagues and visitors part with a sense that they have more to say to each other at a future date rather than the opposite. Build in some 15–30 minute breaks in the day to allow the visitor time to check e-mail, make phone calls, visit the restroom, and so forth. Schedule one meeting of 60–75 minutes with a group of students and/or postdoctoral fellows. Splurge and buy them all lunch or a snack. This atmosphere will foster a dialogue and may leave your younger colleagues with some new insights concerning their own career paths and how to pursue them to everyone's advantage.

You do not need to schedule all of your visitor's time in seminars and formal office settings. Informal time over meals or at unique cultural and natural venues offered by your location (museums, art galleries, parks, concerts, etc.) can be a welcomed surprise for someone from out of town.

If you receive an invitation to present a seminar at another campus or institution, try to go. You never know if your laboratory's next best postdoctoral fellow might turn out to be listening in that audience. Always treat a seminar as an event of critical importance, deserving your full attention and care. Even though you might think of it as just another seminar, your host institution may have a different agenda in mind. They may be using it as an opportunity to evaluate you as a prospective faculty or administrative recruit. Surreptitious interviews are not uncommon in academia, biotech, and large pharmaceutical companies ("big pharma"). Sometimes, you may not even learn that you were being interviewed until later. As they say, do not turn down a job that you have not yet been offered; always put your best foot forward.

REFERENCES

Kirby, D. "Finessing Interviews: Don't Ask, Do Tell." *New York Times*, January 30, 2001.

Kirby, D. "There Are Questions You Shouldn't Answer." *New York Times*, January 30, 2001.

chapter

17

· · · · · · · · · ·

COLLABORATIONS

· · · · · · · · · · · · · · · · ·

The ability to build and maintain good collaborations is invaluable, whether you are in academia or biotechnology. Science is advancing so fast that it is unlikely that any one laboratory alone will command the resources and technologies to fully address any major research question. Consequently, a collaborator in a discipline other than your own can significantly leverage the impact of your research activities and the scope of your conclusions.

STEPS TO FACILITATE COLLABORATION

Some simple proactive steps can facilitate a productive and mutually rewarding collaboration. First and foremost is to establish an atmosphere of respect and appreciation between the principal investigators and the staff. Both parties must share equally in the fruits of their labor. To accomplish this goal, each collaborator should set out his or her goals and expectations at the outset. Discuss in depth potentially litigious issues such as manuscript authorship, grant money allocation, and inventorship on potential patents. Even though some of these issues, like patent inventorship, are predetermined by law, a discussion of these legal aspects in advance by collaborators can prevent unwelcome and unproductive disagreements at a future date. Include institutional level officials in early discussions and talks. For example, if you are submitting a grant application with a collaborator at another institution, make sure the grants offices at both institutions are in communication as early as possible.

Collaborations are as likely to falter in the face of success as in the face of failure. Take steps to prevent any interpersonal issues from arising, both at the principal investigator level and at the level of postdoctoral fellows, students, and staff. It is better to list two postdoctoral fellows as equal contributors to a manuscript than to fight between two laboratories over the first author position on a publication in a prominent journal.

ACKNOWLEDGEMENT

Whenever you give a public presentation of a work, take care to prominently acknowledge your collaborators at the start or conclusion of the talk. Your behavior in collaborations and how others perceive it will influence your opportunities in the future. Science is a small world. Chances are that people will talk to each other about their interactions with you, both positive and negative. Life is a lot easier if you are working with friends instead of working alone and competing everywhere you turn. Even in industry, today's strategic competitor can become a corporate partner in the future. Whenever you can, build your bridges—don't burn them.

18

••••••••

HOW TO CLOSE
A LABORATORY

•••••••••••••••••

All good things come to an end. At some point in your career, you will need to close the doors on your laboratory and move on to greener pastures. Regardless of the circumstances, there are specific steps you will need to take as you carry out this often-bittersweet task. This chapter outlines the specific areas you need to address as you pack up your office and close the door for the last time.

It is important to give the same attention and care to an ending as you do to the beginning. Closure of your laboratory demands the same planning and detail as its opening (see Table 18.1).

Many circumstances can lead to closure of your laboratory. You may have initiated the event by accepting a position at another institution. Alternatively, the event may be prompted by an institutional decision to release your services at the completion of a contract. In academia, this can occur if you have insufficient grant support or have been denied tenure. In biotechnology, it happens routinely due to changes in research objectives or funding issues. In extreme cases, it can reflect the closure of the company itself due to lack of investment and operating capital. Whatever the reason, you can be assured that the process will be an emotional minefield (if not for you, for some of those around you). Regardless, do your best to maintain a professional public demeanor with everyone. In the long run, that will help you sleep better at night.

Table 18.1   Agenda for Closure

Key Considerations

Chemical inventory: Document appropriate disposition and disposal of chemicals.

Biohazard inventory: Document appropriate disposition of biohazards.

Radioisotope inventory: Document appropriate disposition of radioisotopes.

Equipment inventory: Plan how to sell, move, or dispose of it.

Negotiations with institution: Determine how to leave and what to leave and take.

Personnel placement: Consider where the personnel will go next.

Exit interviews: You will interview with the institution and employees.

Once you and your institution have made a decision to part ways, make a plan for how you want to deal with the situation. You may have personal reasons to keep your move private. A company closure event may need to be announced by the board of directors rather than by you or other staff members. Coordinate the announcement of your laboratory's closure after taking such factors into consideration. A public disclosure should be made at the earliest possible date. Before doing so, prepare your closure agenda in as much detail as possible. People do not like change. By presenting a detailed plan to your staff, you will be better able to enlist their continued support and retain your leadership until the conclusion of this phase of your career. No one's interests are served by orchestrating a sense of panic through rumors and premature disclosures of a possible, but by no means definite, change.

After you are certain that your laboratory will close, meet with the appropriate institutional administrators to discuss responsibilities and expectations. These might include your departmental chairman or dean, your company president or CEO, and financial officials. Address the issues listed below regarding the disposition of the laboratory's assets:

1. If you have grants and contracts, determine whether these can and will be transferred with you to your new institution.
2. Finalize dates for processing the grants and for a closure on all outstanding financial obligations. This will require coordination between the grants administration offices at your old and new institutions.
3. Finalize the date when you will physically leave the laboratory and the institution.
4. Determine responsibility for any moving expenses.
5. Address issues relating to health and unemployment insurance for you and your staff. If the umbrella health insurance policy at your company or

university remains intact, you will be eligible for COBRA. This federal mandate insures that you can keep your health insurance policy for at least 12 months by continuing to pay the full cost of your premiums. However, if your company is closing and canceling its health insurance policy, you cannot receive COBRA coverage and will need to take other steps to maintain health insurance coverage for yourself and your family.

6. Determine what vacation and sick leave benefits you will receive at closure. Many institutions require that you work during the final 2–4 weeks prior to your final day of employment. If you have accrued vacation time, you may wish to use it before your departure. Keep in mind that this may be difficult to negotiate, depending on the circumstances of your departure. If you initiate the exit, do not be surprised to face some anger from supervisors or institutional representatives. They may manifest this as a reluctance to authorize approval for a vacation at such a late date. This is just one more reason to use your vacation time as you earn it. Alternatively, if your company has used up its financial resources in a last-ditch effort to secure investment capital, it may no longer be able to honor paid vacation benefits to its staff.

INVENTORIES, CLEANUP, AND INSPECTIONS

A laboratory contains many toxic substances. Institutional, state, and federal regulations require a detailed inventory of these materials and documentation of their safe storage and disposal. Prepare inventories of chemicals, biohazards, and radioisotopes in your laboratory. Arrange for appropriate disposal of all chemicals, biohazardous materials, and radioactive waste. If your company is closing its doors, these will represent a significant (and probably unwelcome) additional expense. Nevertheless, nothing should be left behind. If you are moving chemicals, determine with the mover how these should be packed to meet Department of Transportation and Department of Commerce regulations. Make sure that the empty laboratory is inspected and certified as clean after your departure. This step will protect you from future liability. In a university, the environmental and occupational health services department is likely to perform this function. In many biotech companies renting space, the landlord will contract this process to a private environmental inspection firm. It is in your best interests legally to obtain and comply with such an inspection.

During the laboratory closure, particularly in industry, prepare a document inventory. This can be a set of electronic discs with a complete set of folders for experimental protocols, reports, methods, standard operating procedures (SOPs), manufacturing documents, publications, and patents. A short notebook or table of contents for easy reference should accompany the inventory. This property has great value if you are liquidating a company's assets. It is the permanent record that will allow others to understand and reproduce your work after you have departed. More than anything else, this will be a record of the challenges you faced and the successes you achieved in your endeavors.

EQUIPMENT

Over the course of operation, your equipment has been exposed to chemical and radioactive hazards. Clean and sanitize the equipment and prepare documentation asserting that it is not contaminated in any way. It is advisable to place a sticker on the equipment itself with the date certifying that it has been cleaned. Your movers or anyone acquiring the equipment will need such a document before they can remove it from your laboratory. If your company is closing, you may be liquidating your inventory. If so, determine a value for your equipment and supplies. You can do this from the company's purchasing records or by hiring a used laboratory equipment company to appraise the inventory. Such companies will often buy the entire assets of the laboratory for a lump sum. Often, this recovers less than 10% of the initial value of the equipment items. You may wish to make a photographic record of the equipment items to assist in their presentation to potential buyers. Piecemeal sale of the equipment and supplies may yield a better financial return on the investment. However, it takes time to identify buyers (a luxury you may not have). In biotech, private university collaborators can prove to be an excellent market for used equipment. Unlike public universities, private university purchasing policies are more flexible when they are presented with a unique opportunity for equipment acquisition. Some biotech companies use online auction companies, like eBay (http://www.ebay.com/), to sell equipment during a liquidation or downsizing event.

PERSONNEL

No matter how it happens, you will discover that your laboratory's closure is a shock and surprise to some of your staff. As much as possible, be prepared to support them during this change. This can take several forms. You can offer to prepare letters of recommendation for individuals applying for new positions, either within your existing institution or externally. You can advise them of alternative positions you are aware of that they may wish to apply for. It is recommended that you announce these offers to help when you first publicly disclose the laboratory closure. It is best to make the first announcement of the closure to all members of the laboratory together. Then you can hold additional, one-on-one meetings to address individual concerns.

Everyone in your laboratory is ultimately responsible for his or her own career decisions. As the laboratory leader, you can support employees by providing them with access to your own experience and insights, if it is requested and welcomed. You may be in a position to recruit individuals to a new position, and, if so, it may be appropriate to do this. However, your contract in industry may stipulate that you cannot recruit personnel for a set period of time if you ever leave the company. Nevertheless, no company can restrict an employee from responding to an advertisement from another firm and leaving for career advancement.

There is as much to learn from closing a laboratory well as there is from running it well. Keep your personal interactions professional and constructive until the closure is complete. It is easy to get angry, sad, and scared when a laboratory closes. Try to keep these emotions in check while working constructively with others. You may be surprised to find that the process is rewarding and enlightening. Some of your colleagues may pleasantly surprise you with their positive attitudes and productivity when placed in a stressful situation. Circumstances like these definitely bring out the best in some employees, and these are the people you are likely to remain in contact with after you have all moved on to new opportunities.

chapter

19

•••••••••

PROFESSIONAL EXPECTATIONS OF PHDS IN ACADEMIA AND INDUSTRY

•••••••••••••••••

In your professional capacity, you will need to fulfill the expectations of your superiors. Although the degrees of emphasis on specific performance criteria may differ, both academia and biotechnology share many of the same performance milestones. This chapter reviews these milestones and describes tools you can use to meet them.

Whether you work in academia or biotech, both scientists and administrators will evaluate your performance as a research investigator. Not all of these individuals will have expertise in your field. To maintain objectivity, they will use items such as your publication record, grants, and invited lectures to reach promotion and retention decisions. To keep track of your progress, it helps to maintain a comprehensive curriculum vitae organized around each category (outlined in Table 19.1). You will use this document frequently to summarize and display your accomplishments.

PUBLICATIONS

Nameless (and faceless) administrators and your scientific peers will assess you based, in part, on the number and quality of your peer-reviewed

Table 19.1   Expected Milestones in Academia

Publications	Peer-reviewed manuscripts
	Invited reviews
	Book chapters and books
	Editorials
Grants	Federal
	Private foundation
	State and local
Patents	Pending (national and international)
	Issued (national and international)
Peer review	NIH study section
	Journal manuscript review
	Journal editorial board
Teaching	Didactic (graduate, undergraduate, medical school)
	Graduate student advisor
Community service	University committees
	University and departmental administration
	Mentoring junior faculty
	State and federal scientific committees
	Professional society service
	Organization of scientific meetings
Honors	Scientific awards
	Speaking engagements (university seminar series, meetings, businesses)
Academic freedom	Tenure

publications. Tenure review committees will look at the impact factor of the journals you publish in and the number of times your work has been cited by others in the literature. Many universities set a threshold for the number of publications you need to be considered for tenure and/or promotion in rank. They will note your authorship position (first author, senior author, or contributing author). There will be additional interest in the number of invited review articles and book chapters you have written. Oddly enough, your review articles can turn out to be more widely cited than your primary research articles themselves. Consequently, it is valuable from a career vantage point to take the time to accept invitations to write reviews. These can also provide the opportunity to take a strategic view of the field and to speculate as to its future direction.

GRANTS

Of equal importance to tenure or promotion decisions is your record of grant support. Not all grants are created equal. You will receive more administrative credit and benefit from investigator-initiated grants supported by the National Institutes of Health (NIH) or related federal funding agencies. This reflects the high level of NIH indirect costs. You will receive less benefits at the administrative level for grants funded by federal agencies that mandate lower indirect cost levels; these include the National Science Foundation (NSF), the U.S. Department of Agriculture, and other agencies. Whereas your departmental colleagues will respect grants you receive from national and local private research foundations (such as the American Heart Association, the American Diabetes Association, and the American Cancer Society), administrators will take a somewhat more jaded view. This simply reflects the fact that these grants include low levels of indirect support. Grants from these agencies have their greatest advantage to junior level faculty members who are just starting their laboratories; administrators will be more appreciative of funding from any source during the early years of a career.

There are some exceptions to keep in mind. Occasionally, the NIH and other agencies solicit shared-equipment grants. These generally provide support to institutions for large equipment expenditures if matching funds are provided by a local source (either the university, the state, or another entity). While these are NIH grants, they do not provide any indirect costs; indirect costs are never provided for equipment expenditures. Junior faculty members who have received $1 million in funding on an equipment grant may discover that this has no positive bearing whatsoever during the tenure review process. Consequently, the time and effort for preparing such grants is really a form of community service.

PEER REVIEWING

One measure of career advancement is whether you sit on the other side of the fence with respect to manuscripts and grants. Have you been asked to review submitted manuscripts? If so, by which journals? Are you a journal editor? Have you been asked to review grants by any private foundations or NIH study sections? If so, has this been on an *ad hoc* (one-time) basis, or have you been appointed to the study section roster for several years? All of these matters should appear on your curriculum vitae.

The peer review process is a responsibility and a privilege. Performed correctly, it calls for strict confidentiality. Anything you learn from a submitted manuscript or grant application should not be discussed with anyone other than the journal editor or other members of the study section panel. In addition, you should not communicate your thoughts to the authors of the document directly. Your comments should only be transmitted through official channels.

Whenever you review, remember to treat others the way you would like to be treated yourself. Be prompt in completing your review and submitting it to the journal editor within the defined deadline. You should do your utmost not to let the manuscript get misplaced on your desk or, now that so many submissions are electronic, somewhere in your e-mail folders. Be objective and concise in your comments. If you are going to accept or reject a submission, provide reasons to explain your decision. If you are reviewing a document outside your immediate field of expertise, make sure you are knowledgeable in the background literature. If that is not possible, this is probably a reason to recuse yourself from the review process. It is also appropriate to remove yourself from the review process if you have a conflict of interest or whenever there is the possible perception of one. This includes the review of papers from companies in which you hold a financial interest as well as submissions by faculty members from your own institution, by one of your collaborators, or by one of your former graduate trainees. It may be acceptable to review papers by former postdoctoral fellows who have been away from your laboratory for more than 5 years.

Whenever you write a critique of a manuscript or grant, refrain from any derogatory comments about the work or personal comments about the investigator. These comments are unnecessary and ill-advised; they serve no constructive purpose and do a disservice to the review process itself. Do not ask for any additional experiments that you would be unwilling to support in your own laboratory. In short, be reasonable!

TEACHING

Teaching is a *sine qua non* of academia. In a traditional graduate department, faculty members will be expected to teach one or more classes each term. In a university medical center, expectations for faculty teaching may be reduced. Investigators may only give a few lectures to medical students in one class per year. The demands vary from campus to campus. Your curriculum vitae should include all classes that you have taught, organized, and contributed to; include the years and semesters covered by these activities. There will also be emphasis on the number of graduate and undergraduate students you have mentored. These will include rotating students, students whose thesis committees you were a part of, students who conducted their thesis research in your laboratory, postdoctoral fellows, and even junior faculty members of your department. Your curriculum vitae needs to document their years of training as well as their careers after leaving your laboratory. It is useful to maintain contact with these individuals and to periodically update your records with new information about their career advancement and accomplishments. In some respects, these people represent the most significant product of your career activities and are a legacy of your laboratory.

Despite the number of hours you will expend in teaching, this arena tends to be a secondary consideration in the context of your career evaluation. While students may reward and appreciate excellent teachers, tenure committees may not. Teaching is a necessary but not sufficient criterion for academic promotion in a research institution. In institutions where the major mission is undergraduate education, an investigator's teaching ability and activities will have greater importance. Nevertheless, even if you work in a college rather than university setting, it is important to maintain an active and funded research program.

COMMUNITY SERVICE

Administrators will ask how you have contributed to the academic or institutional community. How have you tangibly demonstrated that you are a good corporate "citizen"? Have you served as a member or chair of committees? If so, which ones? What has been your performance in these capacities? Have you held any administrative positions within the institution (e.g., acting departmental chair) or externally (e.g., officer in a national scientific organization)? Have you performed any state or federal government service (e.g., member of an external advisory panel for the NIH, member of a state-sponsored health related granting agency)? It is very difficult to remember all of these details over the course of your career. Keep track of these items as you perform them.

HONORS AND SPEAKING ENGAGEMENTS

You should also keep a list of any awards you receive in your academic and professional career. This might include induction into an honor society (e.g., Phi Beta Kappa), receipt of a postdoctoral fellowship award from a competitive granting agency, or the selection of your poster at a local meeting as "Best in Show." Keep an updated record of your oral presentations; include the date, location (city, state, country), title, and venue of the occasion (name of the meeting, organization, department and/or institution).

You should place those talks given to nonscientific audiences, such as the Rotary Club or the Lions Club, in a separate section.

ACADEMIC FREEDOM

Expectations cut both ways. If you elect to pursue your career in a university setting, you should receive "academic freedom" as a benefit. This means you should be able to pursue and publish on any legitimate research question as long as you can support the work. You should be free from censorship or restrictions in your scholarly pursuits. As the academic landscape continues to evolve, there are likely to be pressures to curtail academic freedom. This may result from budgetary cuts and/or political agendas at the state and federal legislative levels. If you receive anything less, you should actively challenge these infringements on your contract. This might even mean voting with your feet and moving to a different institution. Under such circumstances, the change will do you good.

BIOTECH INDUSTRY SPECIAL EMPHASES

Industry places greater emphasis on certain expectations than academia does. In biotech, managers use your record of milestone achievements as a measure of your success. Did you meet or beat the corporate milestones and goals assigned to your team each year? Has your effort significantly contributed to the development of a commercially successful product? These objective criteria are a tangible measure of your record in industry but are of far less importance in academia.

PATENTS

In the past, academia placed less emphasis on intellectual property and patents in evaluating life science faculty productivity. In contrast, agricultural and engineering colleges have a long history of encouraging their faculty to pursue patents and of rewarding such efforts. As competition for

Table 19.2   Biotech Industry Emphases
Milestone achievements
Patents
Management skills

research dollars has become more competitive, biomedical research centers are increasingly interested in diversifying their sources of income. Administrators now focus more on their patent portfolios in the life sciences. In some universities, this means that an investigator's record of successful patent applications and licensing has greater significance in the context of tenure decisions and promotion. This also results in a financial return to the investigator. Most universities use licensing fees and royalties as incentives to their faculty. If a patent is successfully licensed, an investigator may directly receive as much as 30–50% of the income from the university.

Your patent record will have greater importance in biotech than it does in academia. Companies fully appreciate the value of patents as a source of immediate and future earnings for their shareholders. In industry, patent productivity is a major criterion for determining the success of a basic research program and of its scientists. Although the basic science investigators in industry rarely command the same direct financial rewards from patents as seen in academia, they do benefit indirectly through the form of bonuses, raises, promotions, and job security. Those investigators who are entrepreneurs and founders of their own companies are the exceptions to this statement.

If you (a) are not involved in a sexual harassment case, (b) do not run your laboratory by the maxim "The beatings will stop when morale improves," and (c) get along reasonably well with your departmental chair and colleagues, it is unlikely that your management skills will receive much scrutiny during an academic tenure review. Industry will place greater emphasis on your ability to manage up and manage down. For example, as a supervisor in a company, administrators will ask whether you and all of your employees have taken the full allotment of vacation time during the year. If not, that speaks poorly for your management skills and ability to run a project smoothly. No single person should be indispensable to the effort; everyone should have time away from the job to refresh themselves and maintain their productivity.

Biotech and big pharmaceutical companies both recognize the role leadership and teamwork play in their long-term success. Consequently, they will provide PhD-level employees with opportunities to study and acquire such skills. It is recommended that you seek out and enroll in any seminars, workshops, or retreats involving management training. These may be time consuming and, at times, uncomfortable. Nevertheless, they will give you skills and tools that can make it much easier to achieve your goals. Include any leadership and management training sessions as a section of your curriculum vitae.

20

PERSONNEL MANAGEMENT SKILLS

This chapter deals with specific personnel management issues that you will face as a senior scientist. You need to be prepared to recruit, hire, mentor, promote, and fire personnel as you advance in your career. Although there may be aspects of these tasks that make you uncomfortable, you cannot run a laboratory without these management skills. This chapter touches on elements of each of these skills.

RECRUITING

As you progress in your career, you will continue to refine your recruiting skills. Recruiting occurs through multiple media, including scientific publications, presentations, advertisements, the Internet, and word of mouth. It is likely that additional modes will become available as the information age progresses; 10 years ago, no one would have considered job-hunting on the computer, but now this is routine. Each method has unique advantages and all are valuable. You should not rely exclusively on a single method. Some recruiting methods are serendipitous, and you should just be thankful for them whenever they arrive. Others count on your network of friends, colleagues, current staff, and collaborators. These people will recommend your laboratory to potential recruits and, hopefully, steer their

---

Table 20.1   Recruiting Scenarios

Word of mouth: Someone in your lab knows someone who is looking for a job **or** someone who knows you has recommended you as a postdoc advisor.

Publications: Someone has read one of your publications and wants to work with you.

Advertisements (scientific publications): Includes the back pages of *Science*, *Nature*, and *Cell*.

Advertisements (local publications): Includes the classified ads in your local paper.

Internet: Someone has visited your laboratory's web site.

Seminar: You meet a potential graduate student or postdoctoral candidate after presenting a seminar at his or her institution.

Fell off the truck: Someone with specific expertise must find a position at your institution due to a spouse's or family move to your area.

---

best students and trainees to you. For certain job categories and in certain institutions, such as state or federal institutions, you will need to hold a position open for a specific length of time after you have placed a public advertisement, usually in the print media.

You can view recruiting from two directions. First, applicants/candidates may seek out your laboratory as a favorable place to continue their careers. Second, you may seek out specific applicants/candidates to address a technical deficit or project need within your laboratory. Often, individual situations prove to be a combination of both. Be prepared to be both the interviewer and the interviewee when you meet with your recruits the first time. Hopefully, you will be able to rely on your former and current staff members to recommend your laboratory environment to future employees.

Hiring

When you want to hire someone, you should spell out in advance what you need and expect from a potential employee. This information is invaluable during the interview process. To provide yourself with maximal flexibility, it is advantageous to have standardized job descriptions on hand for the workforce within your organization. Prepare a generalized list of competencies and skills expected for personnel in various job categories. By having this immediately available, you will be pre-positioned for the applicants who "fall off the truck" and drop into your lap unexpectedly. These documents will also serve as a basis for defining salary ranges within your institution and can facilitate your communication with the human resource management office. You may not even need to go to all of this effort if human resources already has such documents prepared.

You can use your job descriptions as a basis for structuring your interviews and comparing the competencies of individual applicants in an objective manner. Focus your questions around the applicant's experience and skill set as they relate to the responsibilities of the job. There may be particular requirements that you must meet in conducting your interviews. Federal law forbids you from asking specific personal questions (see Table 16.1). You should be prepared to interview a number of applicants, even if the first interview identifies an excellent candidate. Depending on the nature of the organization, you may need to justify why you offered the job to a particular candidate. By systematically addressing the same issues during each interview, you can provide yourself with a rationale to defend your final hiring decision. You will need to document the date, time, length, and location of your interviews as well as conversations you hold with any candidate's references. While such information is not used routinely, you will find it invaluable in those rare circumstances in which someone challenges your hiring decision. Challenges can arise from disgruntled applicants who feel that they were unfairly treated by the interview and recruiting process. While it is less common to face a challenge from within your own organization, this can happen as well.

There are unique hiring situations that can arise. If you are married to another scientist or have a high school or college-age relative who is interested in working with you, you may find yourself facing nepotism regulations. In most organizations, you will not be able to work together with a relative, regardless of the circumstances; both the private sector and most state institutions hold to these rules strictly. Exceptions do occur, but do not count on them. Nepotism can also be an issue when you have the good fortune of recruiting a husband-and-wife scientific team to your institution. You may need to work with your human resource management staff to discover a creative way to bring both employees on board while avoiding the perception of nepotism. Usually, you can accomplish this task by eliminating any situation in which one spouse reports to another. In general, you can save yourself a good deal of grief by working closely with your human resource management office as you go through the process of recruiting and hiring.

MENTORING

If you step back and reflect on your career, you will realize that you have a significant body of experience in your possession. You have learned as

Table 20.2 *Job Description Outline*	
Job title	Generic description of job category (e.g., general lab manager, research associate, or postdoctoral fellow)
Job summary	Who will they report to?
	Who will report to them (i.e., whom will they supervise)?
	What will be their general responsibilities?
Job duties	What are their specific responsibilities? Provide a list.
	What are your expectations with respect to each of these responsibilities? Clearly define what you will require in the way of productivity on the job.
Job specifications	**Required specifications:** Educational background and/or alternative experience. You may wish to make this flexible (e.g., a bachelor's degree with 5 years of experience or a master's degree with 2 years of experience).
	Other factors to be considered: Experience, training, or accomplishments that are desirable in a candidate but not required. You should make this list comprehensive, covering all possibilities to allow yourself maximum flexibility in the future.

much from your mistakes as you have from your successes—possibly more. If you are honest, you will realize that you did not do it all alone. Throughout your training, you had the benefit of mentors who helped guide you through some difficult times. Your mentors were not necessarily the people who told you what to do. More likely, they were the ones who helped you make your own decisions, no matter how difficult they may have been. In some ways, mentors were the people who helped you learn to think for yourself.

Everything comes at a price. Now that you have moved up the ladder and are running your own laboratory, it is time for you to give back to your own junior colleagues. How you do this is up to you. Think back on your own mentors, and try to identify how they helped you. Then incorporate these aspects into your own mentoring style. One way to proceed is to take a personal approach. When a junior colleague comes to you with a problem, resist the temptation to try to solve it directly. Instead, you might relate how you dealt with a similar situation in your own past. Then elaborate on the consequences of your decision, good or bad. Consider taking a Socratic approach. Ask questions to guide your colleague through the situation, allowing the colleague to use his or her own answers to reach a decision. Mentoring will be time consuming. It will be frustrating. It can seem thankless. And, ultimately, it will be rewarding.

Promoting

You may be surprised to learn that your staff members view you with some awe and trepidation. No matter how hard you work to be one of the "guys" or "gals" in the laboratory, they perceive you as having significant power over their careers. And, actually, you do. Administrators within your institution will come to you annually for a performance evaluation of your employees (see Chapter 16 for details on the performance review process). Based on this, you will be asked to recommend members of your staff for raises, promotions, and/or bonuses.

In academia, you will discover that you can give an average salary increase reward of only 3–5% overall each year. So, if you give one individual a 6% raise, you may have to balance it by giving another member of your lab a 0–1% raise. Not an enviable position to be in, is it? Nevertheless, it comes with the territory. Your personnel will invariably discuss their salaries and raises with each other. Even if you plead with staff members to keep their salaries confidential, it would be unwise to expect this to happen. You will need to make a decision on how to handle such situations. While there is no "right" answer on this issue, you should consider two possibilities carefully. The first possibility is running what some might see as a "democratic" laboratory, where all staff members receive the same percentage salary increase. You might think this will alleviate your conscience since you can tell anyone who questions you that everyone received the same proportionate increase. This strategy would be a mistake because you should never respond to questions from one individual regarding the salary of anyone else in your laboratory. This information is confidential, and it would be incorrect for you to divulge it to other employees. It would also be a mistake because unless the members of the laboratory all make the same salary, a percentage increase can still leave the perception of inequities since the take-home dollars in each party's paycheck will differ. Invariably, someone will complain that they did not receive as much money as someone else. In many ways, this option leaves you in a no-win scenario.

Consider an alternative: Do you want to run your laboratory as a "meritocracy," in which all raises reflect your evaluation of the individual's performance? This approach will allow you to recognize those members of your staff who are meeting or exceeding their milestones. This has the potential to maintain or improve their morale and will spur them on to greater achievements. At the same time, you will serve notice to those staff members who are under-performing, letting them know in a tangible way that you are not satisfied with their progress. This can backfire, of course. Individuals passed over for a raise can become disgruntled, complain to colleagues, and fail to maintain their levels of productivity. This can create a negative situation in the laboratory—to put it mildly. Your challenge as a manager will be to use the situation to motivate such individuals. Let them know that improvements in their future performance would be recognized and rewarded. Offer them a detailed plan for how they can achieve success in your eyes through the performance review process (outlined in Chapter 16).

In industry, the size and scope of raises and bonuses is greater than in academia. In addition, if the company is doing well financially, it is possible to give significant raises to all employees who have met or exceeded their milestones. Because industry is more likely than academia to promote teamwork in the laboratory, individuals will quickly learn that their raises and promotions will depend on the efforts and achievements of their colleagues as well as their own. These features allow industry to use the rewards of salary and bonuses more effectively than academia.

For both industry and academia, promotion is rarely a team event. Each individual is evaluated based on his or her accomplishments. Generally, there are specific milestones laid out for moving up a rung on the institution's organizational ladder. Most universities have guidelines for the number of publications, the quality of the journals, and the number and size of the grants expected from a successful candidate. Promotion from assistant to associate professor often coincides with a tenure decision in the basic sciences. In companies, the guidelines may be less well–defined, and promotion may reflect the immediate needs of the company, personnel turnover, and/or a major milestone achievement.

Keep in mind that you can do more to hurt staff members' morale by holding them back than by moving them forward prematurely. The more capable the individual, the more likely he or she is to be actively recruited by someone else (either a competing company or another university). If you wait for your staff member to meet all of your institution's written criteria for promotion, you probably have waited too long. By that point, your staff member may have lost confidence in you, in part because you have failed to show confidence in him or her. Do not be surprised to learn that such individuals have begun to seek out opportunities elsewhere.

As a manager, you will not make the final decision for promotion of a junior colleague. One or more committees, on which you may or may not serve as a member, will be responsible for that decision. While you will have a major say in the matter, your input will not be final. As much as possible, learn how the committee(s) reach promotion decisions within your institution. You will find that this information is valuable not only to your staff but also for yourself.

Terminating

No matter how carefully you screen and train your staff, it is likely that you will face the need to terminate someone's contract. It is never an easy decision and is one that most managers reach reluctantly. Nevertheless, it is imperative that you be aware of the steps involved in the termination process. If you thought you lost sleep when deciding to terminate a position, that is insignificant compared to the trouble you will face if you try to terminate someone and fail.

Employees may need to leave their job for many reasons, including incompetence, unsatisfactory performance, insubordination, inappropriate relationships or contact with fellow employees, breach of confidentiality, dishonesty, or criminal behavior. No matter what the reason, you will need to provide a record of any misconduct.

First, document your expectations of the employee's performance clearly. This document needs to be discussed directly with the employee, and you must provide evidence that he or she has comprehended and acknowledged the job's responsibilities. The document should include a series of milestones with timelines established for their completion.

Second, document the steps taken at the management level to assist the employee in meeting these responsibilities and the goals outlined for performance in the immediate future. You need to give a good faith effort to provide the employee with every opportunity to improve his or her performance rating.

Third, maintain a record of your employee's success (or failure) in achieving the goals and milestones in a timely manner. If any incidents occur during the probationary period, you need to record these in detail and, if possible, list any witnesses who can corroborate the event(s).

Fourth, it is wise to maintain a record of the human resource management office's involvement in the process. This staff can provide witnesses to any meetings you hold with the employee and can give you guidance in how to handle what is likely to be a difficult situation.

During this process, it is likely that the individual will look for an alternative position, either within your institution or elsewhere. You can try to assist the employee in finding a new position; however, if you were terminating the employee, it would be unwise to serve as a reference. This is not in your interest or in the employee's. Follow the institutional guidelines concerning letters of recommendation or reference. At some companies, there is an across-the-board policy prohibiting letters of reference for past employees, regardless of why they left the company. These companies will only confirm the dates of employment and salary records for their former staff. By doing so, the companies seek to avoid any lawsuits arising from either (1) an employee who was dissatisfied with his or her letter of recommendation or (2) another company that felt that an inaccurate letter of recommendation led to its hiring of an inappropriate employee.

The process that has been outlined here is one that you are likely to face in a university or large company. In a small company, it may be different. In many states, contracts will reserve the company's right to terminate employment at will. Under such circumstances, you have the right to terminate an individual's contract on the spot. You may find yourself tempted to do so under extreme circumstances. Remember, though, each action has consequences. It is a small world, and nothing you do will remain a secret. How you treat employees today is likely to influence who you can recruit tomorrow. It is in your best interest to conduct any termination process professionally, resolving it at the institutional level. Do not let the situation evolve into a personal issue between yourself and the employee. While this may seem obvious, it can be difficult to achieve. If you are lucky, you will not have to discover this through personal experience.

21

∙∙∙∙∙∙∙∙∙∙

CHANGING JOBS

∙∙∙∙∙∙∙∙∙∙∙∙∙∙∙∙∙

The scientific workforce has always been transient. In recent years, the length of time anyone stays in a single position or institution has decreased further. Thus, it is likely that you will make a significant change in your career path at least once. This chapter deals with some of the mundane affairs you should consider when making a move.

TRANSITIONING FROM ACADEMIA TO INDUSTRY (AND BACK)

Forty years ago, pharmacology departments were the only life science graduate programs that routinely encouraged their students to enter industry. With the growth of the biotechnology industry and the changing economy, this is no longer the case. Now, cutting-edge research published in *Cell*, *Nature*, and *Science* is just as likely to come from a company as it is from a university. In contrast to many universities, the biotech industry can offer investigators access to unique technology, better salaries, and opportunities to perform high throughput experiments. Consequently, it is more common to see graduate students planning to go directly into industry to pursue their careers. Some make the move early, accepting post-doctoral positions in pharmaceutical or biotech companies. More commonly, people enter industry after completing at least one post-doctoral fellowship in an academic laboratory. Moreover, faculty-level scientists in universities are making the transition to industry later in their careers.

The majority of these individuals discover that the biotech or pharmaceutical environment meets their expectations, and they continue to pursue their careers in the private sector. Nevertheless, some investigators find that they miss aspects of the university environment, including academic freedom, student trainees, or the pleasures of writing manuscripts (and grants!) instead of standard operating procedures (SOPs). Not too long ago, these scientists would be unrealistic in considering a return to academia. They entered industry on a one-way ticket and rarely had the chance to return. Today, this is no longer the case. Many academic departments welcome and actively recruit faculty with industrial experience. Universities recognize that industry offers scientists unique business and intellectual property experience that adds value to its faculty. Professors who have been in biotech or large pharmaceutical companies can develop classroom curricula to train and prepare undergraduate and graduate students for industry and entrepreneurial experiences.

NETWORKING

You may be reading this and thinking that it does not apply to your situation. You are committed to remaining in academia (or industry) and have no desire to change. Regardless, you should develop a network of colleagues, friends, and collaborators in your field who are located in both academia and industry. These individuals can provide you with insights and advice about the two different scientific arenas. More than anyone else, they can help you make a career transition if you choose to do so. Even if you are a tenured faculty member at a university, networks in industry are important. You will have students who desire industry experience. You will be better prepared to mentor these members of your laboratory if you can steer them to scientists you know and respect in companies. Likewise, if you are well established in industry, your networks in academia can provide a pipeline for new employees, new ideas, and potential intellectual property.

INTERVIEWING

If you do investigate a transition from academia to industry, you will face a rigorous interview process. While biotech and pharmaceutical companies are impressed by individuals with strong scientific credentials at all levels, they are looking for employees who can adapt to the unique challenges of industry. This is particularly true if you have been a principal investigator in academia for many years. Industry interviewers want to know if you can relinquish the autonomy you exercised in your university laboratory and become a member of their team. Any company that hires you is making a significant financial investment in your future, and they do not want to lose any money in the process. Table 21.1 presents a partial list of the questions you will face during an industry interview.

No matter what your experience level is, you should view the interview process as a two-way street. Just as you will need to provide information to the company, you should be asking questions as well. Of course, you will want to know about the scientific capabilities of the company. Recognize that there may be features of their research that are proprietary and cannot be divulged unless you have signed a confidentiality agreement with the company.

Table 21.1 *Common Questions Industry Interviewers Will Pose to Academic Investigators*

Are you prepared to:
1. Accept decisions from senior management in a productive way?
2. Drop a promising scientific project for economic or intellectual property reasons?
3. Work outside your current area of scientific interest and expertise if your project is changed?
4. Accept the possibility that you may not be able to report your scientific research at meetings and in publications?
5. Relinquish all your future intellectual property developments to the company?
6. Restrict your employment options for a period of time if you ever leave the company (i.e., agree to not work for any competitors for a period of 1 year or more)?

Do you understand and appreciate:
1. The need to develop a product from your research?
2. The importance of regulatory agencies in your research?
3. The importance of documenting your research in accordance with company policy and forms?
4. The need to interface your research with development programs in the company?

Can you:
1. Become a contributing member of a team?
2. Handle administrative responsibilities within your own program?
3. Develop and pursue patents together with the company's intellectual property attorneys?
4. Accept criticism constructively?

Table 21.2 outlines practical questions that you may not have considered. While these questions may not come up during your first visit with the company, they will need to be addressed before you sign on the dotted line.

Job Title

Job title may appear trivial; it is not. Your title makes a public statement on how you fit into the company's hierarchy. You will discover that this has significant impact on how others perceive you, both internally and externally to the company's environment. Make sure you determine that the title reflects a level of responsibility and seniority that satisfies your expectations. In the best of all worlds, you want to move up as a result of your career transition. While you might accept a lateral move for personal or financial reasons, you should avoid a move backward at all costs. Even if you are in circumstances in which any move seems better than your current situation, avoid the temptation to take any job that comes along. Within a few months, you are probably going to regret the decision.

Resources

The company's scientific resources are critical to your success. Many people discover that they had access to a far richer infrastructure in academia than they can ever obtain in industry. Few companies can rival the technical expertise and equipment available in a major university medical center. Even in those companies that maintain equivalent facilities, their use may be limited due to product-related obligations. Find out specifically what capabilities you will be able to use. If there are techniques or equipment that are missing, find out if you can subcontract these experiments to fee-for-service laboratories in contract research organizations or in university-based core facilities. Do not sabotage yourself by accepting a position in a company where the infrastructure cannot support your project.

Salary

Your salary level means more than just what you will bring home in your paycheck. It is a tangible measure of your value in the marketplace and in your new company. Make sure it is a competitive salary for equivalent positions within the industry. If it is not, you should be asking why. Has the company undervalued your services? Is it trying to obtain your services

Table 21.2	What You Need to Learn During an Industry Interview
Job title	What will be your position title?
	How does this compare to the title of the position you are leaving?
	How does it compare to the title of the people within the company you will report to and supervise?
Resources	What kind of research facilities will you have?
	How does this compare to the space you are leaving?
	What additional company resources will you have access to?
	Will you have access to research resources outside the company?
Salary	What will be your salary?
	Is it calculated on an hourly basis?
	Will there be an opportunity to earn bonuses?
	How does this compare to your current salary?
	How does this compare to the salary of equivalent positions in other companies?
	Will you face a cost of living increase by moving to the company?
Benefits	Will you receive health insurance coverage?
	Will your family receive health insurance coverage?
	Will you receive disability and life insurance?
	Will you have a retirement plan?
	Will you receive paid vacation and sick leave?
	Will you be reimbursed for all travel and business expenses?
Moving expenses	Will you be reimbursed for moving costs?
	Will you need to obtain multiple bids for your move?
	Will you need to use a specific contractor for your move?
	Will you receive any housing relocation costs, such as reimbursement for realtor fees?
	Will you receive short-term housing at your new position?
	Will you be reimbursed for travel and expenses for yourself and your family while house hunting at the new job site?
	Will you be reimbursed for the storage of your property while waiting to move into a new home? If so, for how long?
Stock options	Will you receive stock options in the new company?
	What will be the vesting period?
	What form of stock will you receive?

with the minimum investment possible? Does the offer reflect a weakness in the company's financial resources? Make sure that the salary will compensate you for the risk you are taking by leaving an academic center. Biotech companies depend on venture capital for their financing, and this can be fickle (even in a good economic climate). Will the salary be sufficient to allow you to set aside funds in the event of unemployment?

Benefits

Do not take your benefits package for granted. Small companies with less than 20 employees may not have the resources to provide health insurance, life insurance, or retirement plans to their employees. You should investigate the specifics of your vacation and sick leave policies as well.

Moving Expenses

As a postdoctoral fellow, you may not have received compensation for your move. Do not let that happen again. You should be reimbursed for the cost of moving your personal goods to a new position. If the company does not offer this minimum level of support, you should seriously question its financial stability and/or its corporate policies. In larger companies, you may obtain additional relocation support. Some companies will purchase your existing home and/or reimburse you for realtor fees in the sale of your home. This will help you avoid the logistical problems of holding a mortgage on two properties as you juggle the closing dates on your old and new homes with buyers and sellers. Clearly define with the company's human resource office how many trips they will subsidize for you and your family to look for a new home. If your family will not move with you immediately, determine if the company will reimburse you for expenses while visiting with your family. Find out if there is a limit on the frequency, number, and/or length of such trips. By defining these details in advance with both the company's human resource office and your new supervisor, you will avoid any misunderstandings.

Stock Options

Stock options are one way that companies can compensate you for the risk you face in industry. In a new start-up company, the size of your stock option package should be significantly greater than that of an established company. After all, a new company has no record of success and, without existing products, is unlikely to have a revenue stream. The stock options offered are likely to be based on your salary or your position title. For example, you may receive an offer for half a share to a share of stock for each dollar of your base annual salary. It is likely that the company's board of directors has set aside a specific number of shares and authorized a range of stock options that can be offered to potential employees. Keep this in mind as you negotiate your salary and stock option deal. You will probably reach these discussions in the final stages of your interview. Remember, you can be firm *and* flexible. Salary is something you will realize immediately, whereas stock options are a longer-term and riskier form of compensation. If the company cannot meet your request for one, you can ask for an increase in the other. Good luck!

chapter

22

• • • • • • • • • •

PERSONAL LIFE

• • • • • • • • • • • • • • • • • •

Nearly last, but by no means least, is life outside the job. This book is not so presumptuous to tell you how to lead your personal life; however, it is important to emphasize that this aspect of your life deserves the same attention and care as everything else that has been presented here. You may discover that many of the tools you have used on the job can help you with situations at home and with friends. And the opposite is true as well. Do not be surprised to discover that your 6-year-old child will teach you more about management and supervision than anyone in your workplace ever can. The only question you may have is identifying whether you are managing up or managing down with your child. It will probably be a combination of the two.

CHILD CARE

Children and child care are particularly important issues in the laboratory because of the nature of this type of work. Academia and the biotechnology industry require scientists to be flexible in terms of where they live, causing them to move around the country or the world as frequently as every 2 to 3 years. Often this occurs during an individual's early years of family life and childrearing. Even for individuals who have the good fortune to remain settled in one place, business travel to scientific conferences, meetings with collaborators, and fundraising activities will require them to frequently leave their families for periods of days to weeks. For many families, this presents a significant source of stress.

Since it is uncommon in modern society to have extended family (siblings, parents, cousins, etc.) in close proximity, many scientists have little available support structure in the event of an emergency. Likewise, when both parents in a family are involved in science, they will have to juggle their work responsibilities and ambitions with the demands of their home life. Consequently, when the day care center calls in the middle of a meeting to inform parents of a sick child, one member of the family will need to leave the workplace. Sometimes, individuals will have a trusted friend, neighbor, or employee to whom they will delegate this responsibility; however, experience says that this is the exception—not the rule.

As a manager, you will need to anticipate the child-care-related needs of your employees. By providing your staff with a flexible plan for dealing with such situations, you will improve your staff's morale and productivity. Prepare some mechanism by which staff can take leave time for unexpected child-care emergencies without compromising their work. You may want to allow them to work on weekends or evenings to complete a project that was interrupted during the routine 9-to-5 working day. In addition, be aware that your staff may not be available for frequent travel on the job if they have small children at home. Both spouses and children can be resentful toward the employee and employer before, after, and during a period of extended travel. Do what you can to avoid such situations. For example, schedule business travel for a single day or overnight visit whenever possible.

FAMILY AND FRIENDS

By appreciating the role of family and friends in your life, you will be a better leader and manager for others in your laboratory. Make sure you spend time with family and friends, and encourage your employees to do so as well. This does not need to be divorced from the workplace. In science, it is common to have many close friends and even immediate family in the laboratory. You can hold social gatherings for the members of your laboratory outside of working hours. Informal gatherings at a local watering hole, in a park, or at your home go a long way toward keeping the emotional climate in your laboratory healthy. You will also gain a better appreciation of the people you work with in such settings.

OUTSIDE ACTIVITIES

Likewise, make time for activities outside of work. These can be hobbies, exercise, or anything else you find interesting. Each has the potential to relieve the stresses you will face in running a productive laboratory, either in academia or industry. In particular, exercise is recommended as a worthwhile time investment. As your responsibilities as a leader and supervisor grow, you will discover that you spend a greater number of hours at the computer screen rather than standing at a laboratory bench. Since *homo sapiens* was not designed to be a sedentary animal, you should use regular exercise as a way to maintain your health and well-being. If you are fortunate to belong to an institution with the resources to support a fitness center, you should become a member and encourage your staff members to do so as well. A gym can be a great place for everyone to wind down after a day of work.

chapter

23

·········

PERSONAL DEVELOPMENT

·················

Scientific training promotes and requires a lifetime of learning. There is always a new technology, discovery, or invention around the corner. The same is true in other aspects of your professional life. There is always room for personal growth and development on the job. However, it takes a certain amount of courage and fortitude to achieve this. An individual must be ready and willing to objectively evaluate his or her own areas of strength and weakness. These obviously vary between individuals. Paradoxically, they may also vary within a single person. There are times when your particular character traits prove to be both a strength and an asset. Yet, under different circumstances, these same character traits can be a weakness and obstacle to success.

MICROMANAGING

While this book may appear to be "obsessed" about micromanaging, there is a reason. An education in the basic sciences entrains individuals with a sense of independence and self-sufficiency. Your mentors probably emphasized the importance of performing each step of an experiment yourself and directly monitoring its progress. You were expected to take control and responsibility for the direction and outcome of your studies. Even though this hands-on approach fostered your autonomy, it may also have led to a sense that you could only rely on yourself. If this is true, the consequences of this training may be detrimental to your ability to be effective

Table 23.1   Common Issues in Personal Growth
Micromanaging
Leadership Training
Managing projects and building teams
Teaching
Communicating
Fostering creativity

as a laboratory leader. It is likely to interfere with your ability to delegate responsibility and authority to qualified members of your team. A critical step in anyone's development is to learn how to hand off control to team members. By doing this, you can enhance your productivity dramatically.

LEADERSHIP TRAINING

The book *All I Really Need To Know I Learned in Kindergarten,* by Robert Fulghum, makes a strong case for the role of early socialization experiences in determining behaviors later in life. Business psychologists have written many excellent texts identifying coaches as models for leadership training. There is a fair amount of truth to these arguments. For example, scientists who participated in competitive team sports may have developed coaching skills that benefit them as they run their laboratories. The process of getting a diverse group of individuals to work together toward a common goal is challenging. Often, you will hear investigators describe the process of running their laboratories as being a lot like "herding cats." This section will point out some of the tools that can assist you in making this process more manageable and enjoyable.

Compass

A leader must be able to assess complex situations and deconstruct them into more readily comprehensible components. By doing this, a leader's effectiveness increases exponentially. There are four major "compass points" to evaluate in any situation: data, judgments, emotions, and vision. First, what are the data that have been presented? This is likely to be the area that most scientists are most comfortable in dealing with and accepting. Data consist of the information that everyone involved accepts as real and true; it can be summed up as "just the facts." Second, what judgments have been made regarding that data? Even though everyone may know the data, they may have different opinions about that data. This reflects the judgments they have reached, in part based on their previous experience, speculation, and assumptions. Third, how have the data been expressed and received? This reflects the emotional component of the situation. Finally, where will all of this lead in the future? Ultimately, a leader's role is to present and promote a vision for action and growth that everyone on the team can share and follow. Building consensus around an achievable vision is really what leadership is all about.

Compassion

Before you can deal with others, you have to be able to recognize, understand, and accept your own emotional state. No matter how rational and objective you try to be in a given situation, at some level you also will register an emotional reaction. In the simplest terms, emotion boils down to four states: glad, sad, mad, or scared. People will display one or more of these emotional states, particularly under stressful circumstances. If you maintain a conscious awareness of this fact as you deal with others, it becomes easier to assess the emotional status of your team members. By doing so, you will be better able to interface and communicate with them.

Change

One of the very few things in life you can rely on is that a situation will change. One of the other things you can count on is the likelihood that people will resist that change, whatever it may be, in favor of the status quo. Psychological studies of individuals undergoing extreme life changes have plotted a predictable and reproducible series of reactions (Kübler-Ross, 1969). The initial announcement of a change is met with shock or disbelief. Within a short period of time, this gives way to a sense of anger and/or sadness at the sense of loss. Individuals become scared and may try to bargain or negotiate to avoid the outcome. Failure to do so gives way to a period of depression. Eventually, individuals resolve to accept the new circumstances and move on with their lives.

No matter where you run a research team, you will repeatedly deal with change. This may be the loss of grant funding, the discontinuation of a corporate project, or the graduation and departure of a senior graduate student from the team. Each time you will witness some manifestation of the change paradigm, to varying degrees. Be prepared to look for and recognize the signs in advance. By doing so, you can assist your team in maintaining its equilibrium and focus, particularly in times of stress and uncertainty.

Culture

The tendency of many managers is to recruit employees with backgrounds and behaviors much like their own. With the increasing diversity of cultures and socioeconomic backgrounds within the U.S. scientific workforce, you will quickly discover that the chances are remote for finding anyone resembling yourself in an applicant pool of job candidates. It is important to avoid the trap of harboring any "–isms" in your hiring policies. Most prominent in the public's perception are racism and sexism; however, others to consider are discrimination based on age, socioeconomic class, sexual orientation, and nationality.

Individuals from different generations are likely to view situations from different perspectives. Whereas a new college graduate may see the risk of a start-up biotech company as an exciting, positive component of the job opportunity, a 55-year-old employee is more likely to view this negatively as a threat. Someone who comes from a family in which both parents are college-educated and professional school graduates is likely to approach education differently than an individual who is the first member of his or her family to attend college. In one family, receipt of a graduate education brings an individual closer to his or her parents' own experience; in another family, the same process exposes the individual to a very different career pathway from that of the parents. This may create conflicts for that individual with parents and other relatives whose education went no further than a high school diploma. Each family is likely to hold distinct expectations and aspirations for any professionally trained members of their household. As a manager, you will need to be aware of these potential conflicts and their consequences as they relate to your staff.

An individual's nationality can have a major impact on his or her job. Today, the United States has a greater percentage of first-generation immigrants than any other time in nearly a century. When you deal with an individual for whom English is a second language, you need to take steps to ensure that you communicate clearly and effectively. Take the time and patience necessary to accomplish this task. You may even want to learn the basics of a foreign language. Even if you never become fluent in the language, it will give you a greater sympathy for the challenges your employee faces each day while speaking, writing, and working in an English-only environment. You may also learn revealing aspects of a particular foreign language that explain common mistakes. For example, the Chinese language does not have the same third-person pronouns as English. While

English has words for male (he), female (she), or neutral (it) objects, Chinese has a single word ("ta") for all three. Consequently, it is not uncommon for native Chinese speakers to confuse "he" and "she" when speaking about someone else in English.

Conduct

Scientific training stresses the importance of maintaining a critical and skeptical approach to evaluating all new data and conclusions. The individual scientist's goal is to be objective on the job. This same approach can be destructive when applied to personal relationships and interactions. One step that scientists can use to address this concern is to consciously take steps to express their appreciation to their colleagues more frequently. At first, doing so will feel awkward and unnatural. Nevertheless, as a team leader, you will discover that it does work very effectively. One way to implement this process is to understand that there is a "stroke" (any turn taken by one of the people in a verbal exchange) economy in any conversation. This can be reduced to four basic exchanges: conditional or unconditional positive strokes and conditional or unconditional negative strokes (see Table 25.2).

Conditional strokes relate to a task or tangible achievement, whereas unconditional strokes relate to something that is outside an individual's control. It is helpful to remember the stroke economy while conversing in the workplace, particularly as a manager. For example, there are no circumstances in which an unconditional conversational negative stroke is likely to serve anyone's professional goals. Finding ways to avoid such interchanges is productive and likely to prevent or remove opportunities for conflict in the laboratory.

Canteen

You are going to need a reservoir of tools as you embark on your travels as a scientific leader and manager. One of the most important skills you will

Table 25.2 Examples of Conversational Stroke Economy		
	Conditional	Unconditional
Positive	"You did a perfect job on that report."	"You look great."
Negative	"Your performance on the project was unsatisfactory."	"I hate you."

need is the ability to foster a sense of trust and adventure in your staff. Even though people may have a natural tendency to respond negatively to any changes, you should generate an enthusiasm and willingness among your scientists to "try on" new models or situations with an open mind. One of the most effective ways you can do this is through your choice of language in routine circumstances. For example, consider how you introduce alternatives to your team. You may lean towards an exclusive paradigm, presenting issues to others in an "either/or" framework. At other times, you may be inclusive, presenting issues in the context of a "both/and" paradigm. There are advantages to the "both/and" inclusive model. It does not have an immediate polarizing influence on your audience and has a better chance of stimulating a constructive conversation rather than promoting a defensive posture and destructive argument.

Whenever possible, you should discuss projects and their outcomes without assigning "shame or blame"; such assignment tends to personalize the interchange. It prevents your audience from looking at the data while encouraging them to focus on their emotions. Usually, this evolves into an unproductive scenario. Instead, keep the conversation at a level that promotes a solution to any problems. As the team leader, you can accomplish this by keeping a "self-focus" in the conversation. For example, relate the existing circumstance to similar previous experiences of your own in the laboratory. It takes practice before you can routinely deal with everyday issues in the laboratory in this manner; however, if you can achieve this goal, you will discover that it is an effective tool in facilitating communication with your colleagues and staff.

MANAGING PROJECTS AND BUILDING TEAMS

The application of leadership skills often takes place in the context of individual projects within the laboratory. As you take on and develop specific projects, consider both their "dimensional/mechanical" and "nonmechanical" aspects.

The dimensions and mechanics of a project reflect its environment and resources. To evaluate a project's environment, ask yourself the following questions: What will be the project's goals? What will be quantifiable measures of performance success? Who will sponsor the project? Who will be the project's advocate, either internal or external to the project team? What will be the schedule for intermediate milestones and final completion of the project? Finally, how reliable are the assumptions you have used to define the project environment (i.e., do you need to anticipate any major changes, such as publications from a competing laboratory or company)?

Likewise, resource availability is critical to the project's success. To evaluate a project's resources, ask yourself the following questions: What is the financial commitment to the project (i.e., what is the budget)? What is the level of available expertise and research support, both internal and external to the institution? What facilities will be committed to the project team? Are they adequate to meet the timelines and goals?

The nonmechanical aspects of the project are really the people involved and how they will relate to each other in achieving a common goal. In organizing your project team, you need to define your management structure and process and relate this to everyone involved. How will people communicate (i.e., what is the reporting structure)? Who has authority and responsibility for decisions? It is important to remember that leadership and management are not synonymous. After a project's parameters and plans have been agreed upon, the leader can delegate its implementation to a project manager. The project manager is then charged with leading within the project team. This process is empowering to the staff members and gives them an opportunity to grow their managerial skills through practical experience. It also relieves you from micromanaging the details and routine aspects of the project's operation.

Choosing a project team is challenging. Sometimes you are in a position to advertise and hire specific new recruits based on relevant expertise and experience related to a particular project. More likely, you have an existing pool of talent to draw upon within your organization. As the leader, you need to look at the personality of the team players in addition to their experience and expertise. Not everyone should have the same resume, and, hopefully, they will be professional in their interactions. You need to take into consideration each team member's career objectives, developmental needs, ability to follow directions and accept supervision, and leadership potential. These factors will help you determine how you want to construct your chain of command. One final point to take into account: the sponsor! Ultimately, the team will report its work to some entity. In academia, this might be the National Institutes of Health (NIH). In biotech, it may be a large pharmaceutical company corporate partner or a venture capitalist firm. Regardless, think of the sponsor as a member of your team, and keep it "in the loop." You need to communicate your progress, your success, and your setbacks to them on a regular basis. Failure to do so can derail even the most successful project.

TEACHING

As a leader, you will always be teaching (and learning) on the job. In medical school, much of the clinical teaching is done by the maxim "See one, do one, teach one." While this can be an effective approach, it often devolves into a less efficient model: "See one, screw one up, do one, teach one." Nevertheless, you can learn more from your mistakes than from your immediate successes. It is useful to ask yourself these questions: What were the qualities that you admired most or liked least about teachers you have had in the past? What was distinctive about the most effective (and least effective) teachers you remember? Find ways to emulate and/or avoid those same patterns as you develop your own teaching style.

COMMUNICATING

As a leader, you want your message to penetrate 100% of the "market"— not just the top or bottom 10%. Your job is to find a common ground for collective communication. In graduate school, you probably heard someone say that you should present each slide in a talk three times; first tell people what they are going to see, then tell them what they are looking at, and finally, tell them what they saw. The repetition may be unnecessary for some members of the audience, yet critical for others. People learn and think differently based on educational background, experience, age, and gender. Leaders must always be ready to communicate simultaneously to diverse groups within an audience. For example, whereas some people are auditory learners who best assimilate information through the spoken word, the majority are either visual or tactile learners who use images or hands-on experience to take in new information. To communicate effectively to all of these people in a public address, you will need to present key information through the spoken word, written text, pictures, and diagrams. If the setting is appropriate, you may want to have a hands-on session that allows your audience to touch and manipulate objects or materials related to your topic. It also helps to touch base with your audience to ensure that the message is being transmitted. It never hurts to ask people directly if they have questions or are confused; if they are, take steps to address these misunderstandings so your audience can continue to follow the rest of your presentation.

FOSTERING CREATIVITY

One of the most difficult challenges of scientific leadership is fostering creativity. This book has presented a great deal of information about how to organize facts, people, and tools. Yet scientists rely on creativity to make new discoveries and thrive on the concepts of "spontaneity" and "serendipity." Many scientists will find attempts to develop an "organization" as stifling to the discovery process. How can you, as a leader, reconcile these two apparently conflicting viewpoints?

Some argue that creativity and invention are qualities best displayed by children at play. The most successful scientists are thought to retain this child-like ability to play even as adults. Although you may remember your childhood as a time of freedom, it helps to look back on that period with an adult perspective. At age 4, you could do anything you wanted inside the sandbox as long as no one else got hurt. Your mother did not mind if you built castles, drove trucks, and generally made a mess. While you may not have grown up to be an engineer, the experience did foster your sense of imagination and creativity. Still, your mother did confine the dimensions of your play with rules and physical boundaries. The structure of a laboratory or biotech company serves the same purpose. The key trick is to help your team discover the place within your organization where they can still play creatively in the sand. Even though the adult version of a sandbox is more abstract, it is every bit as important as it was at age 4 to your scientific staff. Find ways to protect this space, and use it to develop novel and innovative discoveries.

REFERENCES

Fulghum, R. *All I Really Need to Know I Learned in Kindergarten: Uncommon Thoughts on Common Things.* New York: Ballantine Books, 1993.
Kübler-Ross, E. *On Death and Dying.* New York: Macmillan, 1969.

INDEX